Essential English for Nurses

An Effective Way to Learn Nursing English

by

Paul F. Zito and Masako Hayano-Zito

看護英会話標準テキスト
学生版

本書の音声教材をダウンロードできます。
1861@nissoken.com
まで空メールを送ってください。

ダウンロードできるコンテンツは，DIALOGUE および EXERCISE 1 の音声です（自己学習用CDと同じです）。

＊EXERCISE 2，EXERCISE 5，KEY WORDS & PHRASES，LET'S MASTER THE DIALOGUE！，LISTENING については，教師用CDにのみ入っています。別途ご購入ください。

Foreword

Effective communication needed in the twenty-first century will rely on people of different cultures who develop creative ways to better understand each other. That is what Paul Zito and Masako Hayano-Zito have successfully accomplished with their popular text entitled *Essential English for Nurses*, in which they provide experiences in health care as the medium for language acquisition. They recognized that nurses and doctors are often called upon to make assessments and diagnoses, and to deliver treatments to their patients who may not speak the same language as the health care provider. In time of health crisis, patients feel so vulnerable and isolated. But, when the patients cannot communicate their concerns because language is a barrier, the crisis becomes even more magnified. The nurses and doctors are also frustrated, especially when the health condition needs to be carefully described for rapid treatment planning.

All of us in the health care field can report incidences that were disastrous because we could not effectively communicate in the patient's language. We vow to do something about it, and look for a simple method of focused learning to help us get ready for the "next time." This organized language learning approach is good, yet a complete approach calls for experiential integration of the language. That is why Zito and Hayano have written their step-by-step vignettes in the vernacular of "how the patient and nurse might really interact." The reality of each situation used in this text is already in the reader's mind because who has not already been the patient, care giver, or family member accompanying the sick person? Learning the English words takes on personal meaning when the learner relives the various situations.

Essential English for Nurses is a "must" tool for any nurse or doctor working in agencies where patients come from different culture and language backgrounds. This text is helpful for the medical and nursing staff who travel abroad and have need to use another health delivery system where English language is the norm. Finally, the interesting situations presented in this book are stimulating for all students in training who wish to be creative in their care, and enter the twenty-first century as effective communicators. The authors have written their text as an outcome of many years in teaching and translating both English and Japanese languages. They are the "intercultural" couple who have traveled and lived in both cultures, and now share their expertise with you.

Thank you for the privilege of reviewing this text. I wish all of you, the readers, great success in using this delightful way to learn the English language in your field.

Annalee Oakes
Dean Emeritus, School of Health Sciences
Seattle Pacific University

序

　21世紀における効果的なコミュニケーションは，異なる文化をもつ人々が，より良い相互理解のための創造的な方法を構築しようとする努力の中から達成されていくことになろう。ジトーポール氏と早野ZITO真佐子氏は，その近著「Essential English for Nurses」において，語学学習の媒体として看護分野における経験を用いながら，このことに見事に成功している。両氏は，医師やナースが，自分達と同じ言語を必ずしも使わない患者に対して，診断や看護診断を下し治療や看護をしていかなければならない立場に置かれ，それに対処するように要求されることがしばしばあるということを十分認識している。本書はその認識の結果である。

　ヘルスケアに携わる私達の多くは，患者の言語を使って効果的に意志の疎通がはかれなかったために問題が起こってしまったという経験を少なからずもっている。そして，この次に対処するために，せめて的を絞った言語学習をしようと誓う。こうしたアプローチはそれ自体はよいのだが，言語を総合的に学習するためには，経験に基づいた言語の統合性が要求される。ジトー，早野両氏が本著の中で，患者とナースの間で実際に交わされる言葉を使いながら，きめ細かいステップ毎の場面設定でダイアログを展開しているのはこのゆえんである。展開されるそれぞれの状況は，すでに読者のよく知るところである。なぜならば，だれもが一度ならずとも患者であったり，介護者であったり，患者に付き添う家族であったりした経験をもっているからである。自分自身の経験がテキストの中で展開される時，その英語学習は個人的に特別な意味をもつことになる。

　「Essential English for Nurses」は，文化的また言語的に異なる背景をもつ患者に対処しなければならない機関で働く医師やナースにとって，まさに必要不可欠の道具となることであろう。また，海外に出かけ英語を基本言語とする医療機関で働こうとする医療関係者にもぜひお薦めしたい。そして，本著のなかで取りあげられている興味深い状況設定は，創造的看護をしたい，効果的なコミュニケーターとして21世紀を迎えたいと願うすべての学生に，大きな刺激となるはずである。本書には，医療関係者や学生に対する教師としての，また日英両言語の優れた翻訳者としての，両著者の長年にわたる専門的知識，見識，経験のすべてが投入されている。両著者は，米国，日本の両文化のなかでの生活を経験し，豊富な異文化交流を基底にもつご夫妻である。

　最後に，本書の監修に携わることのできたことを光栄に思い感謝申し上げるとともに，ご自分の専門分野における英語を，このすばらしい本で学習される皆さま方のご成功を心からお祈り申し上げる。

シアトル パシフィック大学
看護学部 名誉学部長　アナリー・オークス

Preface

In recent years, Japanese nursing professionals have gone abroad for international participation and cooperation in the field of nursing much more frequently than in the past. More nursing students have gone abroad to participate in international nursing studies and conferences. The number of foreign people living in Japan also has increased drastically. It is not unusual anymore to see foreign people living not only in big cities but also in small towns. All of these situations create a growing necessity for people working in the field of nursing to communicate with patients and other nursing professionals who do not speak Japanese. Not every foreign person speaks English as his or her mother tongue. Yet, it is true that the English language makes it possible for more prople in the world to communicate with each other than any other language.

When people living in a foreign culture become sick, they often feel very apprehensive whether, because of language barriers, they can make themselves understood and thereby receive appropriate care. Doctors, nurses, and medical technicians also feel a certain sense of helplessness and frustration in such situations. They too wish they could remove the language barrier that separates them from their foreign patients.

We recently had an opportunity to bring a group of Japanese nurses, nursing students and nursing teachers to an American university for a two-week nursing seminar. All of the attendants of the seminar repeatedly mentioned how they wished to understand and directly communicate with the American lecturers and nursing students whom they met during the seminar.

Thus, knowledge of practical nursing English is essential for Japanese nursing students and professionals to communicate with foreign people studying and working in the field of nursing. It will also become an important skill of theirs when they have to serve the needs of foreign patients whether in Japan or overseas.

When we planned to write this book, we decided to create a textbook that would combine the necessary nursing knowledge and the essential language learning techniques. For ten years, we taught nursing English at Japanese nursing colleges. We were frustrated by the unavailability of a comprehensive and effective English language textbook specifically written for nursing students and professionals. Most of the English language textbooks for nurses in Japan have been written by nursing professionals; while generally excellent in the treatment of nursing situations, they invariably lack what is necessary for English-language study. Since we could not find an adequate textbook, we used to spend a substantial amount of time to prepare supplemental materials before each lesson.

Essential English for Nurses draws upon our many years of experience teaching nursing and medical English to nursing students and doctors at Japanese colleges. The content of the main dialogues is based upon Paul Zito's personal experience as a foreign outpatient and inpatient at Japanese hospitals and medical clinics during his sixteen years of stay in Japan. Therefore, readers of this textbook will find the stories throughout the book very realistic, and they will discover themselves spontaneously learning nursing English.

Each unit is carefully planned, with the main dialogue as its center, so that students may gain a high level of language proficiency in the use of nursing English. Those who study this textbook will gain the necessary proficiency for communication by repeated reading, writing, speaking, and listening to nursing English set out in the text and accompanying CDs. We took an extra effort to create an effective textbook that will satisfy both the learner's interest in nursing and his or her interest in gaining higher proficiency in the English language. We sought advice concerning the details of nursing in Japanese hospital situations from the staff members of Munakata College of Nursing. Dr. Annalee Oakes, then Dean of the School of Health Sciences at Seattle Pacific University, reviewed the whole textbook to make sure that the content was consistent with realistic nursing situations and that the English terminology and expressions were accurately set forth as currently used by American nursing and medical professionals.

We have been active in the various programs enhancing intercultural interactions and understandings in Japan for many years, besides having taught at Japanese colleges. This book has been completed drawing upon these experiences of ours and the knowledge gained from the experiences in both fields, language teaching and intercultural relations. It is our sincere wish that this textbook will help nursing students and professionals effectively learn English in their field and thereby facilitate their competent interaction with English-speaking patients in Japan and overseas.

Language study always requires commitment and effort, and students can expect to experience some frustration and discouragement at times. We hope, however, that they will also experience the joy of communicating with foreign people using their newly acquired skill of the English language. It is our hope that they will someday find the great joy of bringing better nursing care to their foreign patients, which is the result of their improved ability of communication in nursing English. We wish all of you great success with your study.

Finally, we would like to express our deepest gratitude to those who have helped us with our effort to complete this textbook and make it as effective, stimulating, and accurate as possible. So many people have extended their support to us, especially when Paul Zito became seriously ill during the long process of completing this book. Thank you all very much. We feel so blessed to have been able to complete this book in the midst of great love and support from so many people both in Japan and in the United States.

Paul F.Zito and Masako Hayano-ZITO
Seattle, Washington
January 1995

はしがき

　最近は，海外国際協力や海外研修などで，日本の看護関係者が海外に出かけていく機会が増えてきました。また，日本に居住する外国人の数も増える一方で，都会だけでなく，地方の小さな町でも外国人を見かけることが少なくありません。もちろん外国人のすべてが英語を母国語とするわけではありませんが，英語がより多くの外国人とのコミュニケーションを可能にする言語だということは間違いありません。

　外国に住む人は，体調がおかしいとき，それを十分に伝えることができるかどうか，理解してもらえるかどうか，非常に不安を感じ心細い思いをします。医療従事者も，日本語でコミュニケーションできない外国人患者に対するとき，言葉の壁さえなければと戸惑いやいらだちを感じます。また，最近，日本の看護学生，看護学校教師，看護師のグループを米国の大学への研修に引率したのですが，そのとき参加者の間からくり返し聞こえてきたのは，アメリカ人の講師や交流のあった看護学生の話している英語をもう少し自分で理解できれば，少しでも直接話をすることができれば，という多くの声でした。日本国内で外国人患者に対応するにしても，外国で患者に対応したり看護・医療関係者と交流をしたりするにしても，自分の英語力を磨き，さらに専門分野における看護・医療英語の知識を身につけることができれば，自分と相手双方にとって，大変心強い味方を得たことになります。

　今回，この本を執筆することになり，まず念頭においたのは，看護英語の知識と語学学習のテクニックを併せ持つテキストをつくる，ということでした。と申しますのは，長い間看護学生に英語の教鞭をとっていて，この二つをドッキングさせた効果的な看護英語のテキストに出会うことができなかったからです。既刊の看護英語用テキストの多くは，看護専門家によって書かれたもので，看護の知識という点では優れていても，効果的な語学学習という視点に欠けているものが少なくありませんでした。ですから，私たちも授業の度毎に，既刊のテキストに欠けているものを補うべく多くの資料や練習問題を作成し，その準備に膨大な時間を費やしたものでした。

　本著は，十年にわたって工夫を重ねながら看護英語を教えてきた両筆者の経験と知識に基づいて執筆されたものです。また，ダイアログの内容は，ポールジトーが16年の日本滞在中に実際に外来，あるいは入院生活で外国人患者として経験したことが柱となっています。ですから，現実感のあるストーリーを通して違和感なく看護英語を学習していただけることと思います。

各ユニットは，メインダイアログを中心にして，看護英語をステップ毎に，読み，書き，聴き，話すことを繰り返すことにより，学習者が看護という医療分野における総合的な英語力を身につけることができるように組まれています。学習者の看護への興味と英語力向上への興味，その両方を満たすことができるように十分な配慮を加えました。内容の正確さを期すために，日本の臨床現場における実際については，宗像看護専門学校の諸先生方よりアドバイスをいただき，全般的な看護についての内容や米国の看護・医療現場において実際に使われている英語表現などについては，ワシントン州シアトル市のシアトル・パシフィック大学看護学部長（当時，現名誉学部長），アナリー・オークス博士に監修をお願い致しました。

　本著は，長い間異文化交流に力を注ぎ，また日本の看護学校で看護英語教育に携わった者として，少しでも多くの看護学生や実際に看護，医療の現場にいらっしゃる方々の英語力の向上，ひいては看護分野における国際化の一助となれば，との願いをこめて脱稿したものです。語学学習は長い間の努力を要し，苦労もつきものですが，本著を学習する過程において，学習者の方々には，自分の身につけた英語で外国の人々とコミュニケーションをはかることのできる喜びに，ぜひ出会っていただきたいと願っています。そして，外国人の患者に対して，習得した英語でコミュニケーションをはかることができ，より良い看護ができたという喜びをいつの日か味わっていただけることを，筆者として願ってやみません。

　最後になりましたが，よりよい本を完成させたいという願いの中で本著を執筆，脱稿するまでの長いプロセスにおいて，途中ジトーが大病を経験したこともあり，日米両国の本当に数多くの方々から，たくさんの励ましや支え，そしてアドバイスをいただきました。国境を超えた大きな愛の中で，この本の完成を見ることができましたことに心から深く感謝申し上げます。

1995年1月シアトルにて
ジトーポール
早野ZITO真佐子

CONTENTS／目次

UNIT 1　EMERGENCY DEPARTMENT／救急外来

- **DIALOGUE 1**　RECEPTION DESK／受付 ……… 13
- **DIALOGUE 2**　EXAMINATION ROOM／診察室 ……… 18
- **DIALOGUE 3**　GIVING INJECTIONS／注射投与 ……… 23
- **DIALOGUE 4**　EXPLANATION TO A FAMILY MEMBER／家族への説明 ……… 27

UNIT 2　MEETING THE PATIENT／患者との顔合わせ

- **DIALOGUE 1**　SELF-INTRODUCTION AND FIRST MEAL／自己紹介と初めての病院食 ……… 32
- **DIALOGUE 2**　ORIENTATION TO THE WARD／入院病棟の案内 ……… 37
- **DIALOGUE 3**　ASKING HEIGHT, WEIGHT, AND TEMPERATURE／身長，体重，体温をたずねる ……… 42
- **DIALOGUE 4**　OBTAINING THE PATIENT'S HISTORY／患者歴をとる ……… 47

UNIT 3　GENERAL CARE OF PATIENTS／入院患者の全般的ケア

- **DIALOGUE 1**　CHECKING THE PATIENT'S CONDITION／患者の状態をチェックする ……… 53
- **DIALOGUE 2**　BLOOD TEST EXPLANATION／血液検査の説明 ……… 58
- **DIALOGUE 3**　DRAWING A BLOOD SAMPLE／採血 ……… 63

UNIT 4　OPERATION ORIENTATION／手術のためのオリエンテーション

- **DIALOGUE 1**　EXPLAINING ABOUT THE OPERATION: BASIC PROCEDURES／手術についての説明：基本的手順 ……… 68
- **DIALOGUE 2**　EXPLAINING ABOUT THE OPERATION: ANESTHESIA／手術についての説明：麻酔 ……… 72
- **DIALOGUE 3**　TAKING THE PATIENT INTO SURGERY／手術室への搬送 ……… 76

UNIT 5　POSTOPERATIVE CARE／術後のケア

DIALOGUE 1	OBSERVATION AFTER OPERATION（1）／術後観察（1）	81
DIALOGUE 2	OBSERVATION AFTER OPERATION（2）／術後観察（2）	87
DIALOGUE 3	URINARY CATHETERIZATION（1）／導尿管挿入（1）	92
DIALOGUE 4	URINARY CATHETERIZATION（2）／導尿管挿入（2）	97

UNIT 6　PATIENT DISCHARGE／退院準備

DIALOGUE 1	INSTRUCTIONS BEFORE DISCHARGE／退院前の指導	102
DIALOGUE 2	INSTRUCTION ON DIET／食事指導	106
DIALOGUE 3	APPOINTMENT AS AN OUTPATIENT／外来患者としての予約	112

APPENDIX／付録

Parts of a human body／人体模式図（体の部位名）	118
Human organs／人体模式図（器官名）	119
Skeleton／骨格（骨の名前）	121
List of Professionals and Departments in Hospital／診療科や医療職などに関する単語	122
Measurement／度量衡換算表	125

UNIT 1 EMERGENCY DEPARTMENT

🔴 DIALOGUE 1 —RECEPTION DESK

Nurse: What seems to be the problem?

Patient: I sprained my ankle.

Nurse: Which ankle did you sprain?

Patient: My left ankle.

Nurse: When did the injury occur?

Patient: This afternoon.

Nurse: I see. Do you have your health insurance booklet with you?

Patient: Yes, here it is.

Nurse: Mr. Robert, is that right?

Patient: Well, Robert is my first name. My last name is Ordal.

Nurse: Pardon me, Mr. Ordal. Please enter the examination room.

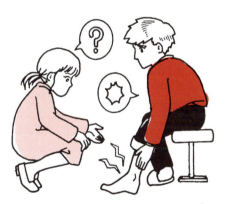

KEY SENTENCES

1. What seems to be the problem?
2. Which ankle did you sprain?
3. When did the injury occur?
4. Please enter the examination room.

KEY WORDS AND PHRASES

Emergency Department
reception desk
sprain
ankle
injury
occur
health insurance booklet（card）
examination room

〔ノート〕health insurance booklet
日本の健康被保険者証は，冊子からカードタイプに切り替わった。カードタイプのものについてはhealth insurance cardと表現した方が適切。

UNIT 1-1

🔴 **EXERCISE 1** —Repeat each sentence in the dialogue after the CD.

🔴 **EXERCISE 2** —Repeat the key sentences.
　　　　　　　　Repeat the key words and phrases.

EXERCISE 3 —Let's learn the key sentences!

　　　　　　上にはKEY SENTENCESで学んだ単語を思い出して入れて練習してください。

> N: What seems to be the _____ ?
> P: I sprained my _____ .
> N: Which _____ did you sprain?
> P: My _____ .

1. matter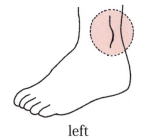
   left

2. trouble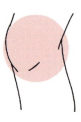
   right

3. problem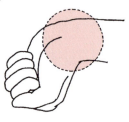
   left

> N: When did the _____ occur?
> P: This _____ .

1.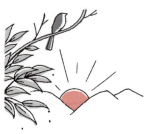

2.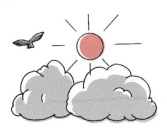

3.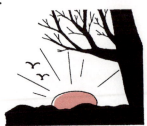

UNIT 1-1

N: Please enter the _____ room.
P: Okay.

1.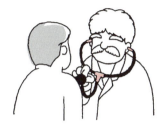
examination

2.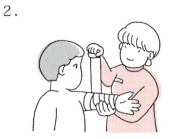
treatment

Master the Expressions!

Fill in the blanks. 空欄を埋めなさい。

N: What seems to be the _____?
P: I _____ my knee.
N: _____ knee did you _____?
P: My right knee.
N: _____ did the _____ occur?
P: This morning.

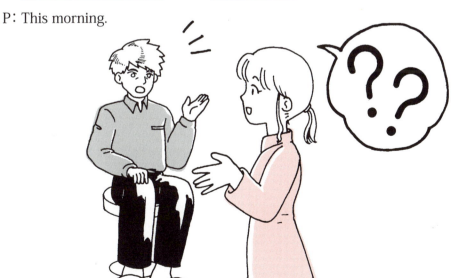

UNIT 1-1

EXERCISE4—First Name? Last Name?

外国人の名前は，姓か名かの区別がつきにくいものです。以下のパターンを使ってその確認練習をしましょう。

_____上にはKEY SENTENCESで学んだ単語を思い出して入れて練習してください。

> N: Mr./Mrs./Miss/Ms. _____ , is that right?
> P: Well, _____ is my _____ name.
>   My _____ name is _____ .
> N: Pardon me, * Mr./Mrs./Miss/Ms. _____ .

*Oh, I'm sorry

1. Susan Schmidt
2. Tom Johnson
3. Diana Silverstein

Spelling & Pronunciation　外国人の名前は発音もスペルもむずかしいものです。

スペルを知りたい時の表現

Would you spell your name for me?

How do you spell your name?

発音を知りたい時の表現

Would you pronounce your name for me?

How do you pronounce your name?

Master the Expressions! ▶

Fill in the blanks.　空欄を埋めなさい。

N: Would you _____ your last name for me?

P: Sure. It's S-I-L-V-E-R-S-T-E-I-N.

N: S-I-L-V-E-R-S-T-E-I-N. How do you _____ it?

P: Silverstein.

N: Silverstein?

P: Right.

N: Thank you, Miss Silverstein.

Let's practice the conversation using the names below!

上のような会話を，以下の名前を使って練習してみてください。

1. David Strand
2. Barbara Howard
3. Richard Ury
4. June Winchester
5. Stewart Caine
6. Gretta Berger

LET'S MASTER THE DIALOGUE!

Now repeat the main dialogue at natural speed with the CD.

LISTENING

What is wrong with each patient? Listen to the CD and make a ✓ under the problem.

CDを聴いてそれぞれの患者の具合の悪い部位に ✓ をつけなさい。

	neck	wrist		ankle		knee	
		left	right	left	right	left	right
1. David Strand							
2. Barbara Howard							
3. Richard Ury							
4. June Winchester							
5. Stewart Caine							
6. Gretta Berger							

UNIT 1-2

DIALOGUE 2 —EXAMINATION ROOM

Nurse： How did you injure your ankle?

Patient： I twisted it while jogging.

Nurse： Your ankle is quite swollen. Are you in much pain?

Patient： Yes, it really hurts when I walk.

Nurse： What kind of pain is it?

Patient： It's a throbbing pain.

Nurse： I see. A physician on call will examine you in a minute.

After the doctor's examination, we'll immediately treat your injury.

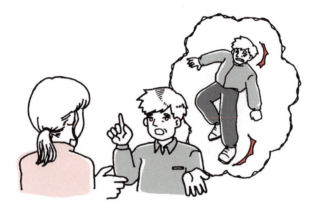

KEY SENTENCES	KEY WORDS AND PHRASES
1. How did you injure your ankle? 2. Are you in much pain? 3. What kind of pain is it? 4. We'll immediately treat your injury.	injure twist swollen pain throbbing hurt physician on call examine examination treat

UNIT 1-2

EXERCISE 1 —Repeat each sentence in the dialogue after the CD.

EXERCISE 2 —Repeat the key sentences.
　　　　　　　Repeat the key words and phrases.

EXERCISE 3 —Let's learn the key sentences!

N: How did you _____ your ankle?
P: I _____ it while _____ .

---

1. injure　　　2. twist　　　3. hurt

jogging　　　exercising　　　playing tennis

N: Are you in much pain?
P: Yes, it hurts _____ .

---

1. a lot　　　2. very much　　　3. quite a bit

UNIT 1-2

> N: What _____ of pain is it?
> P: It's a _____ pain.
> N: We'll immediately _____ your injury.

1. kind
2. type
3. sort

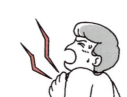
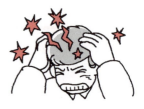

throbbing
treat

stabbing
deal with

splitting
take care of

4. kind
5. type

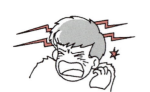
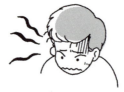

sharp
attend to

dull
look at

Master the Expressions!

Fill in the blanks.　空欄を埋めなさい。

N: _____ did you _____ your wrist?

P: I _____ it while playing volleyball.

N: _____ you in much _____ ?

P: Yes, it _____ a lot.

N: What _____ of _____ is it?

P: It's a sharp pain.

—20—

UNIT 1-2

EXERCISE 4 —Four Steps to Asking About Pain　痛みについてのさまざまな質問

Step 1 : Where?　　Where is the pain?
　　　　どこが　　　Where do you feel the pain?
　　　　　　　　　　Where does it hurt?

Step 2 : How much?　Are you in much pain?
　　　　どのくらい？　Does it hurt very much?
　　　　　　　　　　Do you have much pain?
　　　　　　　　　　How do you describe your pain on a scale of 1-10, 10 being the worst?

Step 3 : What kind?　What kind of pain is it?
　　　　どんな？　　What type of pain are you feeling?
　　　　　　　　　　What sort of pain are you experiencing?
　　　　　　　　　　※kind, type, sortの意味は同じなので、どの文章にも入れ替えて使える。

Step 4 : When?　　When did the pain start?
　　　　いつから？　When did you start feeling the pain?
　　　　　　　　　　How long have you had the pain?
　　　　　　　　　　※１番目と２番目はいつから痛みが始まったかを、３番目はどのくらいその痛みが続いているかその期間をたずねる質問。

Master the Expressions!

Fill in the blanks.　空欄を埋めなさい。

N: Where do you _____ the _____?

P: My neck hurts.

N: Do you _____ much _____?

P: Yes, it's quite painful.

N: What _____ of _____ are you _____?

P: It's a _____ pain.

N: When did the _____ _____?

P: About a week ago.

UNIT 1-2

Let's review again!

痛みについての質問の表現をもう1度復習してみましょう。（　　）の中に与えられた語を文頭，文中あるいは文末に使って，それぞれ3つの文章をつくりなさい。文頭で使う語句には，最初の単語の最初の文字を大文字としている。

Step 1：Where?　　　（1．is　　2．do you　　3．does it）
　　　　（痛みの場所をたずねる）

Step 2：How much?　（1．Are you　　2．Does it　　3．Do you）
　　　　（痛みの程度をたずねる）

Step 3：What kind?　（1．is it?　　2．feeling?　　3．experiencing?）
　　　　（痛みの種類をたずねる）

Step 4：When?　　　（1．When did the　　2．When did you　　3．How long）
　　　　（痛み始めた時期をたずねる）

LET'S MASTER THE DIALOGUE!

Now repeat the main dialogue at natural speed with the CD.

LISTENING

Listen to the CD. Then make a ✓ under the kind of pain and when it started.

1〜4のそれぞれの患者の痛みの種類と痛みの始まった時期について✓で印をつけなさい。

	PAIN					WHEN		
	throbbing	stabbing	splitting	sharp	dull	this morning	this afternoon	three days ago
1								
2								
3								
4								

DIALOGUE 3 —GIVING INJECTIONS

Nurse： We'll need a few x-rays. Please don't move your left foot.
Patient： May I have something to stop the pain?
Nurse： All right. I'll ask the doctor.
Patient： Thanks.
Nurse： （Returns with an injection：） This will relieve the pain.
Nurse： After the x-rays, we'll test for reactions to antibiotics.
　　　　If the results are negative, I'll give you an intravenous injection.
Patient： Why?
Nurse： To prevent any infection.
Patient： I see.

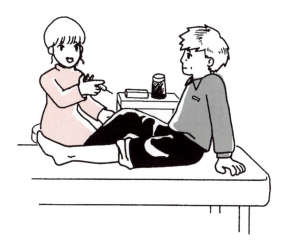

KEY SENTENCES

1. We'll need a few x-rays.
2. This will relieve the pain.
3. We'll test for reactions to antibiotics.
4. I'll give you an intravenous injection.

KEY WORDS AND PHRASES

x-ray
injection
relieve the pain
test for
reaction
antibiotic
result
negative
intravenous injection
infection

UNIT 1-3

🔴 EXERCISE 1 —Repeat each sentence in the dialogue after the CD.

🔴 EXERCISE 2 —Repeat the key sentences.
Repeat the key words and phrases.

EXERCISE 3 —Let's learn the key sentences!

上にはKEY SENTENCESで学んだ単語を思い出して入れて練習してください。

> N: We'll need _____ .
> P: May I have something to stop the pain?
> N: This _____ will _____ the pain.

1. a couple of
2. a few
3. several

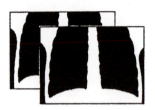
relieve

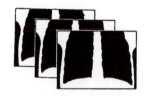
stop

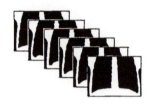
ease

> N: We'll _____ for _____ .
> P: Okay.

1. test
   reactions to antibiotics

2. check
   allergies

3. do a test
   blood type

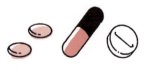

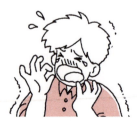

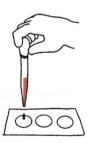

UNIT 1-3

Master the Expressions!

Fill in the blanks. 空欄を埋めなさい。

P: My ankle hurts a lot.

N: I'll _____ you an _____ _____ to _____ your pain.

P: Thank you.

N: After the x-rays, we'll test for _____ to _____ .

EXERCISE 4 — Kinds of Injections 注射の種類

> N: I'll give you a (an)_____ injection.
> P: Why?
> N: To _____ .

1．intravenous 2．intramuscular 3．subcutaneous
　　　　　　　　　　　　　　　　　　　（hypodermic）

　prevent infection　　stop the pain　　reduce the fever

Master the Expressions!

Name the injections. 下線部に注射の種類をあらわす単語を書き入れなさい。

1．A shot into a muscle： _____ _____

2．A shot into a vein： _____ _____

3．A shot beneath the skin： _____ _____

4．An _____ _____ is not so painful, but an _____ _____ really hurts.

UNIT 1-3

💿 LET'S MASTER THE DIALOGUE!

Now repeat the main dialogue at natural speed with the CD.

💿 LISTENING

Listen to the CD and make a ✓ next to what the nurse reported about each patient.

それぞれの患者についての看護師の報告内容と一致するものに ✓ をつけなさい。

1. (　) reactions to antibiotics　(　) allergies　(　) blood type

2. (　) negative　(　) positive　(　) not ready yet

3. (　) an intravenous injection　(　) an intramuscular injection
   (　) a subcutaneous injection

4. (　) prevent infection　(　) stop the pain　(　) reduce the fever

5. (　) 1 x-ray　(　) 2-3 x-rays　(　) 5-7 x-rays

UNIT 1-4

DIALOGUE 4 —EXPLANATION TO A FAMILY MEMBER

Nurse: Mrs. Ordal, did you hear that your husband has a fracture?

Wife: Yes, the doctor told me.

Nurse: He'll need an operation, but please don't worry. He's resting comfortably now.

Wife: That's good to hear.

Nurse: He'll receive our best care while on the Orthopedics Ward.

Wife: I'm relieved.

Nurse: May I have your phone number where we can reach you?

Wife: It's 521-7474.

Nurse: Please come to the reception desk tomorrow morning.

Wife: What do I need to do?

Nurse: You'll need to fill out some forms about your husband's admission to the hospital.

Wife: I see.

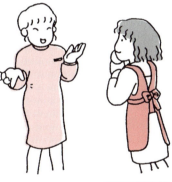

KEY SENTENCES

1. Your husband has a fracture.
2. He'll need an operation.
3. Please don't worry.
4. He's resting comfortably now.

KEY WORDS AND PHRASES

fracture
operation
rest
Orthopedics Ward
forms to fill out
admission to the hospital

〔ノート1〕operation と surgery
ここでは operation を使用したが、通常、手術そのものを指す場合は surgery を使うことが多い。operation には、手術に関わる操作・作業すべてが含まれ、医療以外においても、運営、操作、作業、活動といった意味でも使われる。

〔ノート2〕ward と unit の使い方
通常、大きな病棟は unit を使うことが多い。ward は、1区画がいくつかの専門科の入院患者用に小さく区切られている場合などに用いる。また ward は、4人部屋や6人部屋などの大部屋の病室を指すこともある。

UNIT 1-4

EXERCISE 1 —Repeat each sentence in the dialogue after the CD.

EXERCISE 2 —Repeat the key sentences.
　　　　　　　Repeat the key words and phrases.

EXERCISE 3 —Let's learn the key sentences!

> N: Your husband has a _____.
> W: Yes, the doctor told me.

1. simple fracture　　2. double fracture　　3. sprain fracture

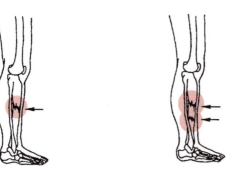 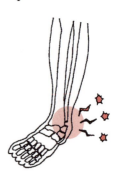

> N: He'll need _____ but please don't _____.
> W: How is he?
> N: He's _____ comfortably now.

1. an operation　　2. surgery　　3. stitches
　 worry　　　　　　be concerned　　be apprehensive

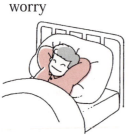 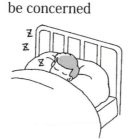 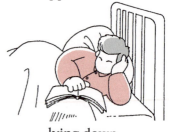

　　resting　　　　　　sleeping　　　　　lying down

> N: Your husband will receive our best _____.
> W: That's good to hear.

1. services   2. care   3. attention

Master the Expressions!

Fill in the blanks. 空欄を埋めなさい

N: Your husband has a _____ _____.
W: Is he in much pain?
N: No, he's _____ comfortably.
W: I'm relieved.
N: Your husband will _____ our best _____.
W: That's good to hear.

EXERCISE 4 — Asking about Phone Numbers　家族の連絡先の電話番号を訊く

> N: _____ I have your phone number where we can _____ you?
> P: Yes, it's 774-3389.
> N: Thank you.

1. May　　　　　2. Could　　　　　3. Can
　 reach　　　　　　 get in touch with　　 contact

UNIT 1-4

More about phone numbers! 電話番号についてのあれこれ

092-541-9921 = 092（area code）＋ 541-9921（local number）

1.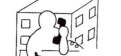
   A: May I have your _____ phone number?
   B: Yes, it's _____.
   A: What's your area code?
   B: It's _____.

2.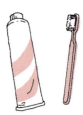
   A: Could I have your _____ phone number?
   B: Yes, the _____ _____ is 093, and the number is _____ — _____. My extension is _____.

Do you know how to say these items in English?

入院時患者の家族に用意してほしい物の名前を，きちんと英語でおぼえよう。

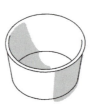

toothbrush & toothpaste

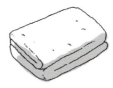

washbasin

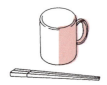

hand towels

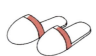

mug & chopsticks

slippers

tissue paper

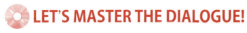

🔴 **LET'S MASTER THE DIALOGUE!**

Now repeat the main dialogue at natural speed with the CD.

UNIT 1-4

🎧 LISTENING

Circle the letter under the picture that accurately reflects the nurse's explanation.

CDの内容と合っている絵に○をつけなさい。

1.
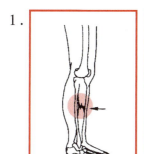
　a　　　　　b

2.
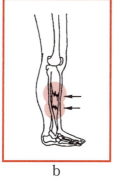 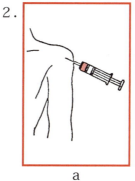
　a　　　　　b

3.
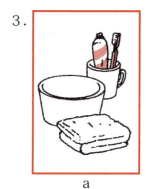 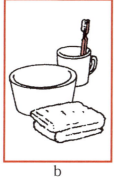
　a　　　　　b

4.
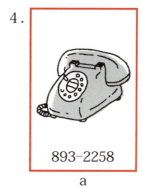 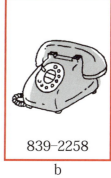
893-2258　　　839-2258
　a　　　　　b

UNIT 2-1

UNIT 2 MEETING THE PATIENT

DIALOGUE 1 —SELF-INTRODUCTION AND FIRST MEAL

Nurse： Good morning, Mr. Ordal. I'm Eiko Yoshida, your primary nurse.

Patient： Nice to meet you, Ms. Yoshida.

Nurse： Nice to meet you, too. How are you feeling?

Patient： Fine.

Nurse： How's your appetite?

Patient： Actually, I'm rather hungry.

Nurse： Good, it's time for your breakfast. Can you eat Japanese meals?

Patient： Yes, but I'd prefer Western food.

Nurse： I understand. I'll tell the nutritionist that you'd like Western-style meals starting tomorrow.

Patient： Thank you.

Nurse： Please bear with the Japanese breakfast this morning.

Patient： Okay.

Nurse： I'll return after breakfast with your medicine.

KEY SENTENCES	KEY WORDS AND PHRASES
1．Nice to meet you. 2．How are you feeling? 3．How's your appetite? 4．It's time for your breakfast.	primary nurse appetite meal prefer nutritionist（dietitian） bear with medicine

〔ノート〕栄養士は nutritionist でも dietitian でもよいが，管理栄養士の場合，registered dietitian（略は RD）で，最近では，registered dietitian nutritionist（略は RDN）を使うこともある。

UNIT 2-1

EXERCISE 1 —Repeat each sentence in the dialogue after the CD.

EXERCISE 2 —Repeat the key sentences.
　　　　　　　Repeat the key words and phrases.

EXERCISE 3 —Let's learn the key sentences!

> N: _____ to meet you, Mr. Keene.
> P: _____ to meet you, too.
> N: How are you?*
> P: _____ .

*Or: How are you doing? ／ How are you feeling?

1. Nice   2. Glad   3. Pleased

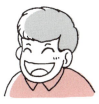
Fine

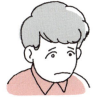
Not so well

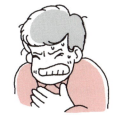
Terrible

> N: How's your _____ ?
> P: It's _____ .

1. appetite today   2. condition now   3. general state of health

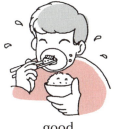
good

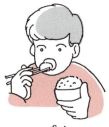
fair

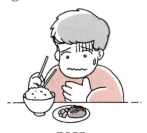
poor

UNIT 2-1

N: It's time for your _____.
P: _____.

1. breakfast 　　2. medicine 　　3. injection

Good 　　　　　Okay 　　　　　All right

Master the Expressions!

Fill in the blanks. 空欄を埋めなさい。

N: Good morning. I'm your _____ nurse.

P: _____ to meet you.

N: _____ to meet you, _____.
　　How are you _____?

P: I'm _____.

N: How's your _____?

P: It's _____.

N: Good. It's _____ for your _____.

EXERCISE 4 —Asking about the Patient's Diet
　　　　　　患者の食事，食習慣についてたずねる

1. Dietary restrictions： 　Are you allergic to any foods?（アレルギー）
　　食事制限について　　　Are you on a special diet?（特別食）
　　　　　　　　　　　　　Do you have any religious dietary restrictions?
　　　　　　　　　　　　　（宗教的理由による食事制限）

—34—

UNIT 2-1

	Possible answers: 考えられる答えの例	Yes. I can't eat eggs and wheat.
		Yes. I'm on a low-sodium diet.
		Yes. I'm a vegetarian.
		Yes. I can't eat pork.
2.	Personal preferences: 日本食に対する 個人的好みについての 質問の例	Can you eat Japanese food?
		Are there any Japanese foods you cannot eat？
		(What Japanese foods would you rather not eat?)
		Do you drink green tea?
	Possible answers: 考えられる答えの例	Yes, but some I can't.
		Yes. I can't eat "sticky soybeans" and Japanese pickles.
		Yes, but I'd prefer black tea.

Let's describe unique Japanese foods!
特殊な日本の食品について説明してみよう！

nattō: fermented soybeans, "sticky soybeans"
umeboshi: pickled plum（s）
oshinko: pickled vegetable（s）
miso: fermented soybean（or rice）paste
konnyaku: cakes（a cake）made from arum root
sashimi: raw fish

〔ノート〕"豆腐"は，少なくとも欧米では"トーフ（tofu）"としてそのまま理解されている。"サシミ（sashimi）"ということばもある程度浸透している。ただし"スシ（sushi）"と言うと"にぎり"と理解されるので，"ちらし"などはrice saladという表現を使ったりもする。

Master the Expressions!

Make questions using the words below.
与えられた単語を使って質問の文を作りなさい。

1. religious / restrictions _____?
2. green / tea _____?
3. allergic / foods _____?

UNIT 2-1

Make matching questions for the answers.

以下が答えとなるような質問の文を作りなさい。

1. _____ ?

   Yes, I'm on a low-sodium diet.

2. _____ ?

   Yes. I can't eat broiled, salted fish.

3. _____ ?

   Yes, but I'd prefer Western-style meals.

🔴 LET'S MASTER THE DIALOGUE!

Now repeat the main dialogue at natural speed with the CD.

🔴 LISTENING

Listen to the CD and circle the correct answer.

CDを聞いてそれぞれの項目で該当する内容を（　　）で囲みなさい。

Feelings	fine okay not so well terrible
Problems	poor appetite pain poor sleep swollen leg
Appetite	good fair not so good poor
Dietary restrictions	low-sodium low-fat no meat no pork
Japanese foods	green tea natto tofu pickled plums

UNIT 2-2

DIALOGUE 2 —ORIENTATION TO THE WARD

Nurse： Let me show you around the ward. I've brought a wheelchair for you.

Patient： Thank you.

Nurse： This is the Nurses' Station. It's staffed twenty-four hours a day.

Mr. Ordal, let me introduce you to our head nurse.

Mrs. Kawada, this is Mr. Ordal, our new patient.

Head Nurse： Nice to meet you, Mr. Ordal.

Patient： Glad to meet you, Mrs. Kawada.

Nurse： The restrooms are down the hall on the right.

The bath and shower rooms are farther down the hall.

Patient： Is there a pay phone on the floor?

Nurse： Yes, it's right before the patients' lounge.

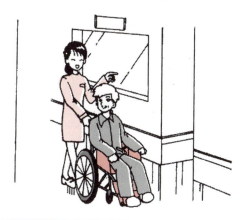

KEY SENTENCES

1．Let me show you around the ward.
2．Let me introduce our head nurse.
3．The restrooms are down the hall on the right.

〔ノート〕アメリカでは，現在は師長の職責のあり方から，head nurseよりもnurse managerを肩書きとして使用する組織が圧倒的に多い。

KEY WORDS AND PHRASES

wheelchair
nurses' station
staffed
head nurse
restroom
bath and shower room
farther down
pay phone
patients' lounge

UNIT 2-2

🔴 **EXERCISE 1** ―Repeat each sentence in the dialogue after the CD.

🔴 **EXERCISE 2** ―Repeat the key sentences.
　　　　　　　Repeat the key words and phrases.

EXERCISE 3 ―Let's learn the key sentences!

　　　　　　上にはKEY SENTENCESで学んだ単語を思い出して入れて練習してください。

> N: Let me _____ you around the _____.
> P: Fine.

1. show　　　　　　2. take　　　　　　3. guide
　 unit　　　　　　　 ward　　　　　　　 hospital

> N1: Let me _____ you to _____ nurse.
> 　　Mrs. _____, this is Mr. Robbins, our new _____.
> N2: Mr. Robbins, _____.
> P: Nice to meet you, too.

1. our head　　　　2. our charge　　　3. your primary
　 Suzuki　　　　　　 Maeda　　　　　　　(use your name)

Master the Expressions!

Fill in the blanks.　空欄を埋めなさい。

N: _____ me _____ you around the hospital.

P: That's great. Thank you.

N: This is the Nurses' _____. Let _____ _____ our head nurse _____ you. Ms. Aritomi, this is our new _____, Miss Somers.

HN: _____ to meet you, Miss Somers.

P: _____ to meet you, Ms. Aritomi.

UNIT 2-2

EXERCISE 4 ─ Directions 方向指示表現

How to go? 行き方を示す（どう行ったらいいのか）

> turn left, turn right, go straight ahead, go up _____ floor (s),
> go down _____ floor (s), go down the hall

turn left　　　　　　　turn right　　　　　go straight ahead

Where is it? 場所を示す（どこにあるのか）

> across from, at the end of, behind, beside, between, close to, on the corner,
> on the _____ floor, on the left, on the right, near, next to

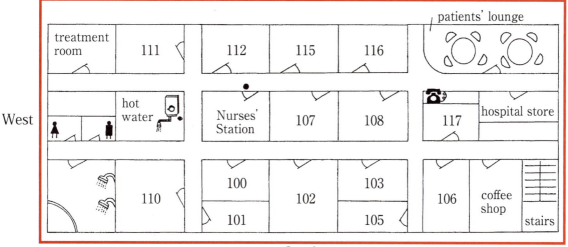

〔ノート〕hospital store
アメリカの場合，病院内の店はgift shopと呼ばれ，取り扱う品物も，ギフト関連商品である。日本の病院のように，患者の日用品を扱うような店はない。基本的に，入院中に患者が必要とするものは，すべて病院で用意するからである。

UNIT 2-2

A patient is asking the following directions standing in front of the Nurses' Station.
(患者は，以下の質問をナースステーションの前でたずねている──•印が患者の位置)

Where is the shower room?	Turn left and then turn right. It's down the hall on the left.
Is there a coffee shop on the floor?	Yes. Go down the hall and turn right. Then turn left. It's between Room 106 and the stairs.

Look at the map on page 39 and fill in the spaces.

前頁の見取図を見ながら，空欄に適切な方向指示表現を入れてみよう。

1. Where is Room 106?   Go _____ the hall and turn _____.
   Go _____ and then turn _____.
   Room 106 is the first room on your _____, _____ _____ the coffee shop.

2. Is there a pay phone on this floor?   Yes. Go _____ ahead.
   The pay phone is ___ the corner, _____ _____ the patients' lounge.

Master the Expressions!

Answer the following questions by looking at the map on page 39.

page39の見取図を見ながら，下のような質問をされた時，きちんとした方向指示ができるようペアで練習してみよう。

1. Where is the hospital store?
2. Where are the stairs?
3. Where is Room 100?
4. Where are the restrooms?
5. Where can I get hot water?

UNIT 2-2

🔴 LET'S MASTER THE DIALOGUE!

Now repeat the main dialogue at natural speed with the CD.

🔴 LISTENING

Listen to the CD and circle the correct location.

以下それぞれの場所に，どう行ったらいいのか，どこにあるのかを，左に挙げた単語が示す場所との位置関係で正しいものを ◯ で囲みなさい。

Restrooms	hallway: on the right on the left in the middle of
Pay phone	lounge: next to across from near
Shower and bath room	hallway: go left and turn right go right and turn left steps: next to close to near beside
Nurses' Station	hallway: at the end of in the middle of
Patients' lounge	floor: end of on the right on the left

UNIT 2-3

DIALOGUE 3 —ASKING HEIGHT, WEIGHT, AND TEMPERATURE

Nurse: What is your height and weight?

Patient: I'm five feet eleven inches and weigh 176 pounds.

Nurse: Do you happen to know the metric measurements?

Patient: No, I'm sorry I don't.

Nurse: I'll calculate into centimeters and kilograms later.

　　　　Let's take your temperature.

　　　　Please place this thermometer under your arm.

Patient: All right. (A few minutes later：) It looks like 37.5 degrees.

Nurse: (Takes the thermometer：) You have a slight fever.

　　　　Normal body temperature is 37 degrees centigrade.

Patient: I felt slightly feverish.

Nurse: I'll make a temperature conversion chart for you.

Patient: That would be helpful.

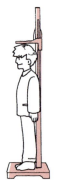 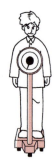 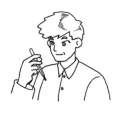

KEY SENTENCES

1. What is your height and weight?
2. Please place this thermometer under your arm.
3. You have a slight fever.

KEY WORDS AND PHRASES

metric measurements
thermometer
degrees
fever
feverish
normal body temperature
centigrade
conversion chart（table）

〔ノート〕アメリカでは医療や科学などの専門職を除いては，十進法の度量衡であるメートル法が使われていない。重量・長さ・温度などの単位が，他の大多数の国とは異なっているため，アメリカ人に対しては，このユニットで示すような換算が必要になってくる。

UNIT 2-3

🔴 **EXERCISE 1**—Repeat each sentence in the dialogue after the tape.

🔴 **EXERCISE 2**—Repeat the key sentences.
　　　　　　　Repeat the key words and phrases.

EXERCISE 3—Let's learn the key sentences!

_____ 上にはKEY SENTENCESで学んだ単語を思い出して入れて練習してください。

> N: What is your _____?
>
> P: It's _____.
>
> N: Do you know what that is in _____?
>
> P: Let me see. It's _____?

1. height 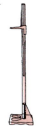　　2. weight 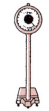　　3. temperature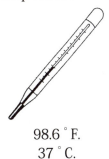

　　6 ft. 2 in.　　　　185 lbs.　　　　98.6 °F.
　　188 cm.　　　　　83.8 kg.　　　　37 °C.

Do you know how to convert?　換算の仕方を知っていますか。

Length:　1 in. = 2.54cm.; 12in. = 1 ft.　　Liquid:　1 oz. = 29.573cm^3
（長さ）　1 ft. = 30.48cm.　　　　　　　（液体）　1 pint = 0.473L

Weight:　1 lb. = 453g　　　　　　　　　　　　　1 quart = 0.946L
（体重）　1 oz. = 28.349g　　　　　　　　　　　1 gallon = 3.7853L

Temperature:　C. = centigrade／Celsius（摂氏），F. = Fahrenheit（華氏）
温度換算
（華氏と摂氏）　freezing point: 0°C. = 32°F.

　　　　　　　boiling point: 100°C. = 212°F.

　　　　　　　(_____ °F. − 32) × 5 ÷ 9 = _____ °C.

　　　　　　　_____ °C. × 9 ÷ 5 + 32 = _____ °F.

UNIT 2-3

> N: Please place this _____ under your arm.
> P: It looks like _____ degrees.
> N: Yes, you have a _____.

1. 37
   normal temperature

2. 37.5
   slight fever

3. 39
   high fever

Master the Expressions!

Fill in the blanks. 空欄を埋めなさい。

N: What's your _____ ?

P: It's 5 feet 9 inches.

N: What's your _____ ?

P: 187 pounds.

N: Now place this _____ under your _____.

P: All right.

N: It's 38.7 degrees. You have a _____ _____.

P: What's that in Fahrenheit?

N: It's _____ degrees.

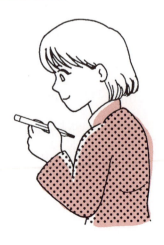

UNIT 2-3

EXERCISE 4—Descriptions of Physique　体格の表現

height（身長）

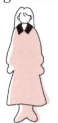 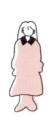

tall　　medium height　　short
　　　　average height

weight（体重）

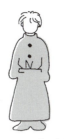 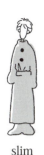

heavy set　　average build　　slim
　　　　　　　　　　　　　　slender
　　　　　　　　　　　　　　thin

［用例］

・She is average height and weight.
・She is of average height and weight.
・He is heavy set.
・He is slender.

小さくて細い人の場合：She is petite.

医学的な問題があるように肥満している人の場合：He is obese.（肥満はobesity）

ガリガリに痩せている場合：He is so thin. She is so skinny.

Master the Expressions!

Describe the four persons below.

上の表現を使って下の患者たちの体つきを述べてみなさい。

1．Nancy Sanchez　　2．Tom Wells　　3．Mary Jenkins　　4．Bill Durrell

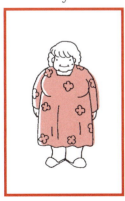 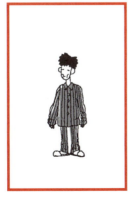 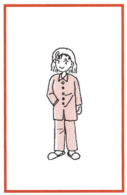 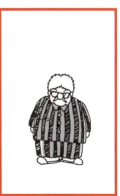

UNIT 2-3

🔴 LET'S MASTER THE DIALOGUE!

Now repeat the main dialogue at natural speed with the CD.

🔴 LISTENING

Listen to the CD and circle the correct answer.

CDをきいて，それぞれの項目で該当するものを（　　）で囲みなさい。

Height in ft.	6′2″	6′4″	6′	6′6″
Weight in lb.	115	150	155	105
Height in cm.	183	138	180	188
Weight in kg.	86	68	66	88
Temperature C°	36.4	36.7	37.5	37.6

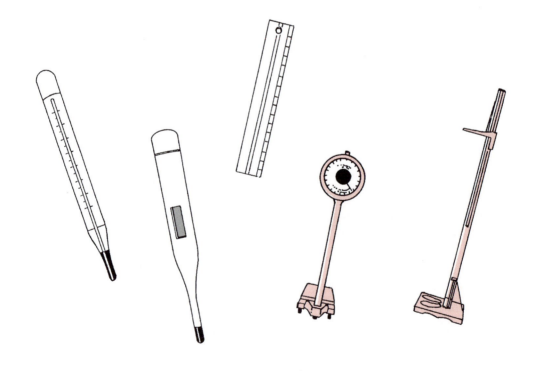

DIALOGUE 4 —OBTAINING THE PATIENT'S HISTORY

Nurse: Mr. Ordal, we'll need a few personal details for our records.
Patient: Okay.
Nurse: What is your occupation?
Patient: I'm a music teacher.
Nurse: Are you allergic to any foods or medicines?
Patient: No, I'm not.
Nurse: What is your general state of health?
Patient: I'm in good health, but sometimes I have high blood pressure.
Nurse: Do you have any headaches now?
Patient: No.
Nurse: Let's take your blood pressure. Please extend your right arm.
Patient: What is my BP?
Nurse: It's 120 over 80. It's normal.
Patient: That's good to hear.

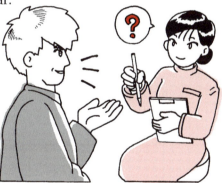

KEY SENTENCES

1. What is your occupation?
2. Are you allergic to any foods or medicines?
3. Let's take your blood pressure.

KEY WORDS AND PHRASES

occupation
be allergic to
general state of health
high blood pressure
headache
extend
BP (blood pressure)

UNIT 2-4

🔴 **EXERCISE 1** —Repeat each sentence in the dialogue after the CD.

🔴 **EXERCISE 2** —Repeat the key sentences.
Repeat the key words and phrases.

EXERCISE 3 —Let's learn the key sentences!

　　　　上にはKEY SENTENCESで学んだ単語を思い出して入れて練習してください。

N: What _____?
P: I'm a (an) _____.
N: Where do you work?
P: I work for _____.

1. is your occupation　　2. kind of work do you do　　3. do you do

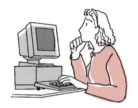
computer programmer
ABC Software

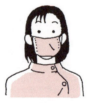
dental hygienist
Dr. Robert Miller

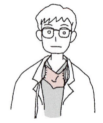
engineer
M&P Company

N: _____ to any foods or medicines?
P: Yes. I'm _____ to _____.

1. Are you allergic　　2. Do you have any allergies　　3. Do you have any allergic reactions

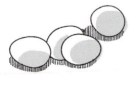
eggs

milk

penicillin

UNIT 2-4

> N: Let's take your _____.
>
> P: Okay.
>
> N: Your pressure is _____ over _____.
> _____.

1．120 / 80

　It's normal

2．90 / 54

　You have low
　blood pressure

3．170 / 110

　You have high
　blood pressure

More Expressions about Blood Pressure!　血圧関係の表現をもっと学ぼう！

Abbreviations： blood pressure →BP

　　　　　　　　high blood pressure →HBP

　　　　　　　　low blood pressure →LBP

Expressions：

HBP： You have high blood pressure.　　　LBP： You have low blood pressure.

　　　You have hypertension.　　　　　　　　　You have hypotension.

　　　You are hypertensive.　　　　　　　　　　You are hypotensive.

Your pressure is 120 over 80. → 120 / 80 mmHg（筆記の場合）
　　　　　　　　　↓　　　↓
　　　　systolic pressure　diastolic pressure

blood pressure manometer：an instrument to measure blood pressure
（hemodynamometer）

Master the Expressions! ▶

Fill in the blanks.　空欄を埋めなさい。

N： What is your _____？

P： I'm a tennis instructor.

N： Are you _____ _____ any foods?

P： Yes, I'm _____ _____ wheat.

UNIT 2-4

N: Now let's _____ your _____ _____.

　Please _____ your right arm.

P: Okay.

N: It's 130 _____ 85.

EXERCISE 4 —Aches, Pains, Soreness　いろいろな痛みについての表現

> N: Do you have a (an) _____?
> P: _____ , _____.

1．headache　　　　2．earache　　　　3．backache

Yes, sometimes.　　No, I don't.　　Yes, all the time.

The Five Aches: 以下の5つの体の部位については，そのすぐあとにache（痛み）という単語をつなげて，その部分の痛みの名前とすることができる。

backache
earache
headache
stomachache
toothache

→ 1．I have a (an) _____.
　　↓
2．I have a pain / an ache in my _____.
3．My _____ hurts / aches.

Aches and Pains: その他の部位の痛みについては以下のような表現をとる。

1．I have a pain / an ache in my _____.
2．My _____ hurts / aches.

UNIT 2-4

Soreness: 筋肉や皮膚に関連する痛みの時に使う。

throat（喉の痛み）
1．I have a sore throat.
2．My throat is sore.

other soreness（その他の痛み）
1．My _____ is sore.（筋肉痛）
2．The patient has a bedsore.（褥瘡）
3．She has a cold sore.（口辺ヘルペス）

〔ノート〕bedsore
bedsoreはいわゆる床ずれ。専門用語としては，decubitus（褥瘡）やpressure ulcer（圧迫潰瘍）を使う。

Master the Expressions!

Write the name of the pain next to the line.（　　）の中に痛みの名前を書きなさい。

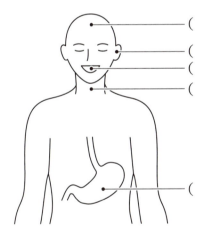
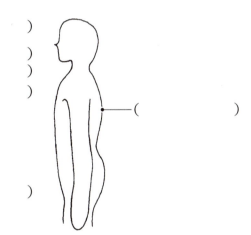

〔ノート〕pain
painは、可算名詞と不可算名詞がある。局部的な痛みについては、例えば「背中に痛みがある」という場合、I have a pain in my back. と可算名詞を使い、pain にはaを付ける。しかし「痛みがありますか？」と部位を限定しないで質問する場合は、Do you have any pain? と不可算名詞として使いaを付けない。

UNIT 2-4

Fill in the spaces with ache, pain, sore, or hurt.

以下の空欄にache（s），pain，sore または hurt（s）のいずれかの単語を入れて文を完成させなさい。

I have an _____ in my right arm.

My right arm _____ .

I have a _____ throat.

My throat is _____ .

I have a _____ in my stomach.

My legs are _____ .

🔴 LET'S MASTER THE DIALOGUE!

Now repeat the main dialogue at natural speed with the CD.

🔴 LISTENING

What are John Stevens's personal details? Listen to the CD and fill in the details on his chart.

患者ジョン・スティーブンズについて以下の内容を聞き取り，個人ファイルを完成させなさい。

Patient's Name：	John Stevens
Occupation：	
General state of health：	
Blood pressure：	
Allergies：	

UNIT 3 GENERAL CARE OF PATIENTS

DIALOGUE 1 —CHECKING THE PATIENT'S CONDITION

Nurse： Are you having difficulty using crutches?

Patient： No. It was a bit awkward at first, but I'm accustomed to them now.

Nurse： Good. Are you sleeping all right?

Patient： No. Sometimes I have to use the bathroom and can't get back to sleep.

Nurse： I'll ask the doctor to prescribe a mild sleeping pill.

Patient： All right.

Nurse： Are your bowel movements regular?

Patient： Yesterday I had diarrhea but not today.

Nurse： How many times did you pass urine yesterday?

Patient： Let me think. Probably six times.

Nurse： How is the pain in your ankle?

Patient： I don't feel much pain now.

Nurse： That's good to hear.

KEY SENTENCES

1. Are you having difficulty using your crutches?
2. Are you sleeping all right?
3. Are your bowel movements regular?
4. How many times did you pass urine yesterday?

KEY WORDS AND PHRASES

crutches
prescribe
mild
sleeping pill
bowel movement
diarrhea
urine

〔ノート〕crutches
松葉杖は通常2本ペアで使うことが多いので，ここでは複数形crutchesとしているが，1本だけの場合はもちろんa crutchという表現となる。

UNIT 3-1

🔴 **EXERCISE 1** —Repeat each sentence in the dialogue after the CD.

🔴 **EXERCISE 2** —Repeat the key sentences.
　　　　　　　Repeat the key words and phrases.

EXERCISE 3 —Let's learn the key sentences!

　　　　上にはKEY SENTENCESで学んだ単語を思い出して入れて練習してください。

> N: Are you having _____ _____ ing _____?
> P: _____.
> N: That's not good.（Oh, I'm sorry.）/ That's good.

1．use crutches　　　2．pass urine　　　3．adjust to hospital life

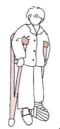　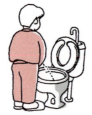　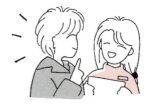

　Yes, somewhat　　　　Sometimes　　　　　I'm doing okay

> N: Are you _____ ing all right?
> P: _____.

1．sleep　　　　　　2．eat　　　　　　　3．feel

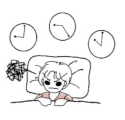　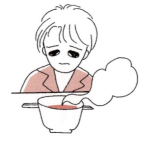　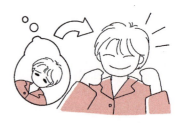

I have difficulty　　I have no appetite　　Better than yesterday
falling asleep

UNIT 3-1

N: _____ your _____ regular?
P: _____.

1. bowel movements   2. sleep   3. headaches

   No, they're irregular   I'm not sleeping well   They don't seem to go away

N: How many times did you _____?
P: _____.

1. pass urine yesterday   2. get up to use the restroom last night   3. wake up because of the pain

   I don't remember   Once   Twice, I think

Master the Expressions!

Fill in the blanks. 空欄を埋めなさい。

N: Any problems using your _____?

P: No, actually I can walk with them quite well.

N: Are you _____ all right?

P: Yes, I even had a nice dream last night.

N: Great. Are your _____ _____ regular?

P: Yes, they are.

N: Good. How many times did you _____ _____ yesterday.

P: Four or five times, I think.

UNIT 3-1

EXERCISE 4 —Urination and Bowel Movements
排尿と便通についてたずねる

1. Irritation or inflammation： Is urination painful?
   痛みや炎症について
   Are you having difficulty urinating?
   Do you have any pain when you urinate?
   Do you feel any burning sensation with urination?

2. Abnormalities： Is the urine cloudy?
   排泄物の異常について
   Have you passed any black stools?
   Have you passed any blood?

3. Changes in Regularity： Are you constipated?
   定期性の変化について
   Are your stools loose?
   How often do you urinate daily?
   Would you like a laxative?

Master the Expressions!

Make questions using the words below.

左の語を使って，排尿，排便についてたずねる文章を作ってみましょう。

1. cloudy： _____ ?
2. constipated： _____ ?
3. pass blood： _____ ?
4. black stools： _____ ?
5. urinate daily： _____ ?
6. medicine for constipation： _____ ?

UNIT 3-1

💿 LET'S MASTER THE DIALOGUE!

Now repeat the main dialogue at natural speed with the CD.

💿 LISTENING

Listen to the CD and place the number in the box matching the patient's condition.

CDを聞き，それぞれの症状を訴えている患者は左の誰か番号を記入しなさい。

1. Mr. John Brandon   (　) frequent urination
2. Ms. Pat Wong   (　) blood in the stools
3. Mrs. Judith Roberts   (　) cloudy urine
4. Mr. James Hunter   (　) pain with urination
5. Miss Andrea Lee   (　) constipation

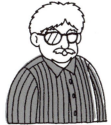
Mr. John Brandon

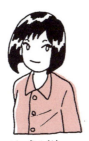
Ms. Pat Wong

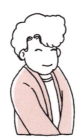
Mrs. Judith Roberts

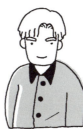
Mr. James Hunter

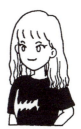
Miss Andrea Lee

UNIT 3-2

DIALOGUE 2 —BLOOD TEST EXPLANATION

Nurse： Mr.Ordal, tomorrow morning I'll need a blood sample for some tests.

Patient： Why is a blood test necessary?

Nurse： We'll need to do a complete blood count to check for anemia and liver function.

Patient： I see.

Nurse： I'll be here for the sample at six o'clock tomorrow morning.

Patient： Six in the morning! Why so early?

Nurse： We need the sample before you've had breakfast.

Patient： Okay, I understand. How much blood will you need?

Nurse： About 20 cc from your right arm. That's normal for a CBC. You won't feel any aftereffects.

Patient： Am I going to have any other tests tomorrow?

Nurse： No, no other test. You can rest quietly afterward.

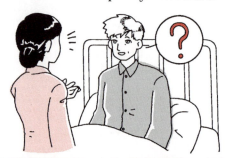

KEY SENTENCES

1. I'll need a blood sample for some tests.
2. We'll need to do a complete blood count to check liver function.
3. You won't feel any physical aftereffects.
4. You can rest quietly afterward.

KEY WORDS AND PHRASES

blood test
blood sample
complete blood count（CBC）
liver function
anemia
aftereffects

〔ノート〕checkとcheck for
check for ～は,「～があるかどうかを調べる」という意で, checkは「～を調べる」である。したがって「貧血があるかどうかを調べる」はcheck for anemiaで,「肝機能を調べる」はcheck liver functionとなる。

UNIT 3-2

🔴 **EXERCISE 1** —Repeat each sentence in the dialogue after the CD.

🔴 **EXERCISE 2** —Repeat the key sentences.
Repeat the key words and phrases.

EXERCISE 3 —Let's learn the key sentences!

> N: We'll need a _____ for some tests.
> P: Why is it necessary?
> N: To check for/check _____ .

1. blood sample   2. urine specimen   3. throat culture

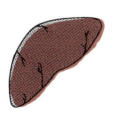
anemia

kidney function

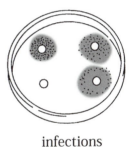
infections

> N: We'll need to do _____ to check _____ .
> P: When will you know the results?
> N: _____ .

1. a CBC
   liver function
2. a urinalysis
   your kidney function
3. an ultrasound
   for any tumors

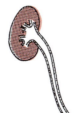
Tomorrow

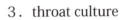
In a few days

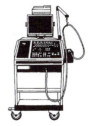
Immediately

UNIT 3-2

N: You won't feel any _____.
P: _____.

1. physical aftereffects　　2. discomfort whatsoever　　3. side effects

　That's good to hear　　I'm relieved to hear that　　Thank goodness

N: You can _____ afterwards.
P: I was afraid I'd have some _____.
N: No, you don't have to worry.

1. rest quietly　　2. relax comfortably　　3. eat regularly

　aftereffects　　　　discomfort　　　　dietary restrictions

Master the Expressions!

Fill in the blanks. 空欄を埋めなさい。

N: Ms. Silver, We need to do a _____ _____ _____ to check your _____ function.
P: How much blood do you need for the _____?
N: About 20 cc.
P: I hope I won't be dizzy afterwards.
N: It's a normal amount for a blood test. You won't feel any _____ _____.
P: That's good.
N: You can _____ quietly afterwards because we won't have any more tests today.

EXERCISE 4 — Testing Different Body Functions

体の部位別にいくつかの検査名も覚えておこう。

Brain	脳	MRI (magnetic resonance imaging)	磁気共鳴断層撮影
		CT (computed tomography)	CTスキャン
		electroencephalography	脳波検査法
		EEG (electroencephalogram)	脳波，脳電図
Liver	肝臓	ultrasound (ultrasonography)／ultrasonogram	超音波（超音波検査法）／超音波検査図
		CT (computed tomography)	CTスキャン
Heart	心臓	stress test	ストレス検査
		electrocardiography	心電図検査（法）
		EKG／ECG (electrocardiogram)	心電図
		angiocardiography	血管心臓造影（法）
		angiography (angiogram)	血管造影（図）
Lung(s)	肺	x-ray	レントゲン
		CT (computed tomography)	CTスキャン
Kidney(s)	腎臓	ultrasound (ultrasonography)／ultrasonogram	超音波検査（法）／超音波検査図
		CT (computed tomography)	CTスキャン
Abdomen	腹部	endoscopy	内視鏡検査
		upper endoscopy	胃鏡検査（カメラ）
		colonoscopy	結腸鏡（大腸内視鏡）検査
		sigmoidoscopy	Ｓ状結腸内視鏡検査
		x-ray (stomach) using barium sulfate	胃透視（バリウム）
		ultrasound (ultrasonography)／ultrasonogram	超音波検査（法）／超音波検査図
		laparoscope (laparoscopy)	腹腔鏡（術）

UNIT 3-2

Master the Expressions!

Write the name of the test for the organ in the parentheses.

（　　）の器官の検査をするのに必要な検査名を空欄に入れ文章を完成させなさい。

We'll need a _____ test.（heart）

Tomorrow we'll do an _____ .（liver）

This morning you'll have an _____ taken.（heart）

Today you're scheduled for a _____ .（brain）

We'll take you now for an _____ .（brain）

LET'S MASTER THE DIALOGUE!

Now repeat the main dialogue at natural speed with the CD.

LISTENING

Note：BB＝before breakfast, AB＝after breakfast, Aft＝afternoon

上記の略記号に気を付けて，CDの内容に合っているものを◯で囲みなさい。

Michelle J. Walker						
	\multicolumn{3}{c}{Types of Tests}	\multicolumn{3}{c}{Time of Test}		
1st Test	CT	CBC	MRI	BB	AB	Aft
2nd Test	blood	ultrasound	urinalysis	BB	AB	Aft
3rd Test	EEG	EKG	CT	BB	AB	Aft

DIALOGUE 3 — DRAWING A BLOOD SAMPLE

Nurse: Good morning, Mr. Ordal. How are you this morning?

Patient: Fine, but I'm still sleepy.

Nurse: Sorry to wake you up so early. Please roll up your sleeve.

Patient: Okay.

Nurse: Let me tie this rubber tubing around your arm. Now make a fist with your thumb tucked in.

Patient: All right.

Nurse: Do you feel any tingling in your fingertips?

Patient: No.

Nurse: All right. We're finished. You can relax now.

Patient: That was like a pinprick. My arm is hardly bleeding.

Nurse: I've had lots of practice. Now press this cotton to your arm and bend it up.

Patient: Okay. Thank you.

Nurse: Here, let me place this adhesive patch on the puncture site.

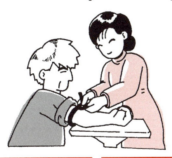

KEY SENTENCES

1. Please roll up your sleeve.
2. Now make a fist with your thumb tucked in.
3. Do you feel any tingling in your fingertips?
4. You can relax now.

KEY WORDS AND PHRASES

roll up
rubber tubing (tourniquet)
make a fist
with one's thumb tucked in
tingling
fingertip
pinprick
bleeding
adhesive patch
puncture site

UNIT 3-3

EXERCISE 1 —Repeat each sentence in the dialogue after the CD.

EXERCISE 2 —Repeat the key sentences.
　　　　　　　Repeat the key words and phrases.

EXERCISE 3 —Let's learn the key sentences!

> N: Please _____ your _____.
> P: Okay.
> N: Now make a _____ with your _____ tucked in.

1. roll up／sleeve　　2. extend／right arm　　3. stretch out／left arm

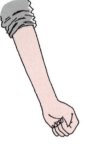　　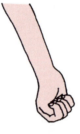　　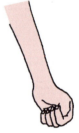

　　fist thumb　　　　　　grip thumb　　　　　　fist thumb

> N: Do you feel any _____ in your _____ ?
> P: _____.

1. tingling／fingertips　　2. tension／chest　　3. soreness／arm

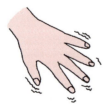　　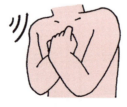　　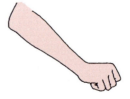

　　Yes, I do　　　　　Quite a bit, actually　　　Not anymore

UNIT 3-3

> N: You can _____ _____.
> P: All right.

1. relax now   2. breathe normally   3. rest comfortablly

Master the Expressions!

Number the sentences in the order of occurrence. Then practice the situation of drawing blood using the following sentences with a partner.

下の文を患者に指示，質問する順に並びかえ番号をつけなさい。次にペアになって下の文を使って採血の場面を練習しましょう。

( ) You can relax now.
( ) Make a fist with your thumb tucked in.
( ) Please roll up your sleeve.
( ) Press this cotton to your arm.
( ) Do you feel any tingling in your fingertips?

EXERCISE 4 — Compound Words Using Blood   bloodを使った熟語あれこれ

WBC	white blood cell; white blood count	白血球，白血球数
RBC	red blood cell; red blood count	赤血球，赤血球数
pl.ct.	（blood）platelet；（blood）platelet count	血小板，血小板値
plasma	（blood）plasma	血漿
serum	（blood）serum	血清
gas analysis	blood gas analysis （O_2/ CO_2/ pH）	血液ガス分析 （酸素/二酸化炭素/水素イオン指数）
loss	blood loss	出血，失血
clot	blood clot	血餅，血栓

UNIT 3-3

culture	blood culture	血液培養
coagulation	blood coagulation	血液凝固
cells	blood cells	血球
sugar	blood sugar	血糖
vessel	blood vessel	血管
volume	blood volume	（全）血液量
transfusion	blood transfusion	輸血

Master the Expressions!

Fill in the spaces with the correct word.

下記の空欄に，前頁で学習したことばの中から最も適切なものを入れ，文章を完成させなさい。

1. The liquid part of blood that separates from the clot is the _____.
2. The formed elements of blood consist of the _____ cells, _____ cells, and the _____.
3. A great loss of blood requires a blood _____.
4. When blood thickens after bleeding it is called _____.
5. The total amount of blood in a person's body is blood _____.
6. A tubular part of the body that carries blood is a blood _____.
7. The analysis of O_2, CO_2 and pH in the blood is called blood _____.

LET'S MASTER THE DIALOGUE!

Now repeat the main dialogue at natural speed with the CD.

UNIT 3-3

🔴 **LISTENING**

Listen to the CD and circle the letter under the picture that accurately reflects the nurse's explanation.

CDを聞いて正しい内容を示している絵の下の記号を ⬚ で囲みなさい。

1.
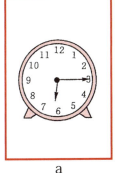

a   b

2.
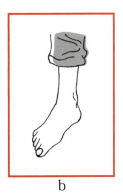

a   b

3.
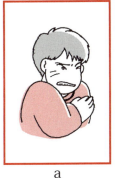

a   b

4.
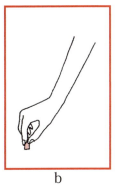

a   b

〔ノート〕 さまざまな血管などの名称

動脈	artery	静脈	vein
動脈圧	arterial blood pressure	静脈圧	venous pressure
大動脈	aorta	大静脈	large vein (vena cava)／cava
冠動脈	coronary artery	深静脈	deep vein
頸動脈	carotid artery	中心静脈	central vein
肺動脈	pulmonary artery	中心静脈圧	central venous pressure
末梢血管	peripheral vessel	毛細血管	capillary (blood) vessel

UNIT 4 OPERATION ORIENTATION

DIALOGUE 1 —EXPLAINING ABOUT THE OPERATION : BASIC PROCEDURES

Nurse: Good morning, Mr. Ordal. I'm a surgical nurse for your operation. How are you feeling today?

Patient: Good morning. I'm feeling fine.

Nurse: I've come to explain about your operation tomorrow afternoon.

Patient: I'd appreciate that.

Nurse: In the morning a nurse will shave and disinfect your leg. Next you'll receive an enema to clear your bowel.

Patient: What about breakfast?

Nurse: You can't eat or drink anything on the day of the operation. Instead, you'll receive an IV solution.

Patient: How long will the preparations take?

Nurse: Only a couple of hours. After you change into a surgical gown, you'll be taken on a gurney to the Operating Room.

Nurse: Oh, here's your breakfast. I'll come by later to continue my explanation.

KEY SENTENCES

1. I've come to explain about your operation.
2. You'll receive an enema to clear your bowel.
3. You'll be taken on a gurney to the operating room.

KEY WORDS AND PHRASES

surgical nurse
operation
shave
disinfect
enema
bowel
IV solution
surgical gown
gurney
operating room (OR)

UNIT 4-1

🔴 **EXERCISE 1** ─Repeat each sentence in the dialogue after the CD.

🔴 **EXERCISE 2** ─Repeat the key sentences.
　　　　　　　Repeat the key words and phrases.

EXERCISE 3 ─Let's learn the key sentences!

　　　──── 上にはKEY SENTENCESで学んだ単語を思い出して入れて練習してください。

> N: How are ＿＿＿＿＿ ＿＿＿＿＿ ing?
> P: Fine, thank you.
> N: I've come to ＿＿＿＿ about ＿＿＿＿＿＿＿＿＿＿.
> P: I'd appreciate that.

1. you / feel　　　　2. you / do　　　　3. things / go

   the hospital regulation　your test results　your operation

> N: You'll receive ＿＿＿＿ to ＿＿＿＿ your ＿＿＿＿.
> P: Does it hurt?
> N: Not a bit.
> P: Good.

1. an enema　　　　2. a laxative　　　　3. an IV solution

   clear / bowel　　take care of / constipation　reduce / fever

〔ノート〕operationとsurgery
外科手術の場合operationでもsurgeryでも同義で使われるが，現在はsurgeryの方がより一般的。手術室はoperating roomという表現が一般的である。operationは，機械などの操作，ある作業の実施などの意味でも使われる。

UNIT 4-1

P: What will happen next?
N: You'll be taken on a (an) _____ to the _____.
P: I see.

1. gurney   2. wheelchair   3. ambulance

Operating Room   X-ray Department   main hospital

Master the Expressions!

Fill in the blanks. 空欄を埋めなさい。

N: Good morning. How are you _____?

P: Not bad.

N: I've come to _____ about your surgery.

P: Okay.

N: After you change into a surgical gown, you'll _____ an _____ to clear your bowel.

P: Does it hurt?

N: Not a bit. Then you'll be _____ on a _____ to the Operating Room.

P: I see.

EXERCISE 4 —Disinfection and Sterilization 消毒と滅菌

消毒，滅菌に関する語いを覚えよう。(発音と意味)

1. disinfection (n)　消毒（病原体の殺菌）
   disinfect (v)　消毒する
   disinfectant　消毒薬

2. sterilization (n) 　　滅菌（全微生物の殺菌）
　　sterilize (v) 　　　滅菌する
　　sterile (a) 　　　　滅菌した
　　sterilizer 　　　　 滅菌器
　　sterile solution 　 無菌溶液
　　sterile water 　　　滅菌水
　　sterile gauze 　　　滅菌ガーゼ

〔ノート〕disinfectとsterileの違い
disinfect: 有害な菌を殺菌，あるいは減少させるプロセスを意味する。
sterile: すべての微生物を完全に殺すことを意味する。

LET'S MASTER THE DIALOGUE!

Now repeat the main dialogue at natural speed with the CD.

LISTENING

Listen to the dialogue. Then listen to the questions about the dialogue and choose the correct answers below.

対話を聞きなさい。次に対話についての質問を聴き，正しいものをa．b．c．の中より選び（　　）で囲みなさい。

1. a. in the morning of the surgery
   b. one day before the surgery
   c. right before the surgery
2. a. to see how things are going
   b. to inform of the patient the operation procedure
   c. to give the patient an IV solution and an enema
3. a. a little later than usual
   b. a little earlier than usual
   c. as usual
4. Put the numbers in the correct sequence.
   対話の内容に沿う順に番号をつけなさい。

_____ The patient will be taken on a gurney to the Operating Room.

_____ The patient will change into a surgical gown.

_____ The patient will receive an enema.

_____ The patient will receive an IV solution.

UNIT 4-2

DIALOGUE 2 —EXPLAINING ABOUT THE OPERATION : ANESTHESIA

Nurse: You'll receive a spinal anesthetic before the operation. Your lower body will be completely anesthetized.

Patient: Will I be conscious during the operation?

Nurse: Yes, but you'll feel absolutely no pain during surgery.

Patient: How long will the operation last?

Nurse: About two hours. Afterwards, we'll wheel you into the Recovery Room.

Patient: I see. What will you do there?

Nurse: We'll monitor your postoperative condition and make sure you're stable.

Patient: How long will I be there?

Nurse: Not very long. When your condition stabilizes, you'll be brought back to your room.

Patient: I understand.

Nurse: Do you have any questions?

Patient: Well, I can't think of anything at the moment.

Nurse: In that case, I'll see you in the Operating Room tomorrow.

Patient: Thanks for stopping by.

KEY SENTENCES

1. Your lower body will be completely anesthetized.
2. We'll monitor your postoperative condition.
3. When your condition stabilizes, you will be brought back to your room.

KEY WORDS AND PHRASES

anesthesia
spinal anesthetic
be anesthetized
conscious
surgery
recovery room
postoperative condition
stabilize

UNIT 4-2

EXERCISE 1 — Repeat each sentence in the dialogue after the CD.

EXERCISE 2 — Repeat the key sentences.
Repeat the key words and phrases.

EXERCISE 3 — Let's learn the key sentences!

上にはKEY SENTENCESで学んだ単語を思い出して入れて練習してください。

> N: You'll receive a spinal anesthetic.
> P: What will happen to me?
> N: Your lower body will _____ completely _____.
> P: I hope I won't feel any pain.
> N: Don't worry. You won't.

1. anesthetized　　2. numbed　　3. senseless

> N: After the operation, you will be taken to the Recovery Room.
> P: What will you do there?
> N: We'll _____ your _____ there.
> P: I see.

1. monitor　　2. check　　3. observe

　postoperative condition　　general condition　　recovery from the surgery

> P: What will happen next?
> N: When your _____, you will be brought back to your room.
> P: I see.

1. condition stabilizes　　2. condition is stabilized　　3. condition is stable

UNIT 4-2

Master the Expressions!

Fill in the blanks. 空欄を埋めなさい。

N: You will receive an _____ before the surgery.

P: What kind?

N: It will be a _____ _____ .

P: Does it anesthetize my whole body?

N: No. Only your _____ body will be _____ .

P: Am I _____ during the operation?

N: Yes, but you won't feel any pain. After the surgery, we will take you to the _____ Room.

P: What will happen there?

N: We'll _____ your _____ condition.

EXERCISE 4 ─ Anesthesia　麻酔について

麻酔の種類や関係する語い，表現を学ぼう。音読して発音を学ぼう。

1. Types of anesthesia:　general anesthesia　　全身麻酔
   麻酔の種類
   　　　　　　　　　　　spinal anesthesia　　脊椎麻酔
   　　　　　　　　　　　epidural anesthesia　硬膜外麻酔
   　　　　　　　　　　　local anesthesia　　　局所麻酔

2. anesthetic ── anesthesia ── anesthetize

   anesthetic (n): You will receive an anesthetic before the operation.
   麻酔剤

   anesthesia (n): The operation will be done under anesthesia.
   麻酔

   anesthetize (v): Your whole body will be anesthetized.
   麻酔をかける

—74—

UNIT 4-2

Master the Expressions!

A．麻酔の種類を（　）の中に記入しなさい。

Your lower body will be anesthetized.　（　　　　　　　　　）

Your whole body will be anesthetized.　（　　　　　　　　　）

Your left thumb will be anesthetized.　（　　　　　　　　　）

B．（　）の中に適切な語を記入しなさい。

P: Will I receive an（　　　　　）for my arm before the surgery?

N: Yes. Your surgery will be done under（　　　　　）.

P: Will my whole body be（　　　　　）?

N: No. You'll receive only a（　　　　　）（　　　　　）.

P: Then, I will be conscious during the surgery?

N: Yes, but you won't feel any pain.

LET'S MASTER THE DIALOGUE!

Now repeat the main dialogue at natural speed with the CD.

LISTENING

Listen to the dialogues. Then listen to the questions about the dialogues and write the correct answers in a few words.

CDの会話を聴き，会話についての質問に数単語で答えなさい。

	PATIENT 1	PATIENT 2	PATIENT 3
QUESTION 1			
QUESTION 2			
QUESTION 3			
QUESTION 4			

UNIT 4-3

DIALOGUE 3 —TAKING THE PATIENT INTO SURGERY

Nurse: Mr. Ordal, we're taking you into surgery now.

Patient: I feel slightly drowsy after receiving that injection in my shoulder.

Nurse: You were given a tranquilizer to relax you physically and mentally. There's no need to worry.

Patient: My mouth is dry, and I'm really thirsty.

Nurse: That's an aftereffect of the injection. We can't give you anything to drink, so please bear with it.

Patient: Can I gargle?

Nurse: All right. (A gurney is brought for the patient.) It's time to transfer you from the bed to the gurney.

Patient: (After gargling：) I feel slightly dizzy.

Nurse: Can you move by yourself?

Patient: Not easily.

Nurse: Here, let me help you.

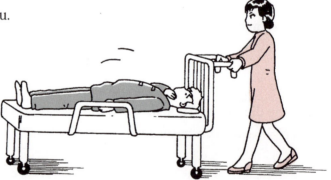

KEY SENTENCES	KEY WORDS AND PHRASES
1. We're taking you into surgery now. 2. You were given a tranquilizer to relax you. 3. Can you move by yourself? 4. Here, let me help you.	drowsy tranquilizer physically and mentally thirsty gargle transfer dizzy

UNIT 4-3

🔴 **EXERCISE 1** —Repeat each sentence in the dialogue after the CD.

🔴 **EXERCISE 2** —Repeat the key sentences.
　　　　　　　Repeat the key words and phrases.

EXERCISE 3 —Let's learn the key sentences!

　　　_____ 上にはKEY SENTENCESで学んだ単語を思い出して入れて練習してください。

> N: Mr. Smith, are you _____?
> P: Oh, is it time to go?
> N: Yes. We're _____ you into _____ now.
> P: I hope everything goes all right.
> N: Don't worry. It will.

1. ready　　　　2. all set　　　　3. prepared

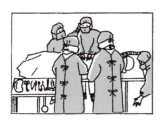　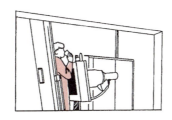　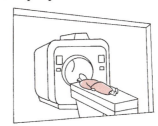

the Operating Room　　the X-ray Room　　the MRI Room

> P: I feel slightly _____.
> N: You were given a _____ to _____.
> P: Oh, I see.
> N: You'll feel better in a while.

1. sluggish　　　　2. drowsy　　　　3. sleepy

　　sedative　　　　pain reliever　　　　tranquilizer
　　calm you down　　ease your headache　　relax you

UNIT 4-3

> N: Can you _____ by yourself?
> P: Not really.
> N: Here, _____.
> P: Thank you.

1．walk　　　　　2．move　　　　　3．use it

Master the Expressions!

Fill in the blanks. 空欄を埋めなさい。

N: Mrs. Andrews, we're _____ you _____ surgery.

P: All right, but I feel slightly drowsy.

N: You've been given a _____ to relax you.

P: I feel a little dizzy too.

N: _____ you move by _____ ?

P: I'm not sure.

N: Here, _____ me _____ you.

P: Thank you.

EXERCISE 4 —*Gaman shite kudasai* 「我慢してください」

医療現場では，痛みや不快を伴う治療も多い。

患者の不安を受け止めながら，つらい時にも我慢していただくための表現を学ぶ。

以下の会話をペアになって練習してみよう。

1．P: I hate injections.

　　N: Well, this might hurt a bit, but <u>please bear with</u> me.

　　P: Please do it gently.

　　N: Yes, of course.

2．P: I'm so hungry.

　　N: I'm sorry, but you can't have anything until the anesthetic wears off completely.

P: When will that be?

N: In a couple of hours.

P: Two hours!

N: I'm sorry, but please be patient.

3. N: Well, Mr. King, I have to ask you a lot of questions. Please put up with me.

    P: How many are there?

    N: About thirty.

    P: Well, that's sure a lot.

4. N: This treatment can be very painful, but please endure.

    P: Don't worry. No matter how painful it is, I will endure it to get well.

    N: Good for you! That's the attitude.

〔ノート〕我慢する
put up withとbear withの場合，そのあとに必ず誰に対して，あるいは何に対して我慢するのかその対象としての目的語を必要とする。be patientの場合，be patientのままでも使用できるし，be patient with＋目的語という表現にしてもよい。

Master the Expressions!

Write a correct word on each line so that each sentence will mean *gaman shite kudasai*.

全体が「我慢してください」という意味になるように適切な単語を下線上に一語ずつ記入して，対話を完成させなさい。

1. N: You have to keep your body still in here for about one hour.
    Please be _____.

    P: I'll try.

2. N: You must have the IV for two hours. Please _____ _____ _____ it.

    P: All right.

3. N: When the anesthetic wears off, you will experience some pain for a while.
    Please _____ _____ it.

    P: I guess I have to.

UNIT 4-3

4. N: You'll have to go through several tests today.

   I hope you can _____ .

   P: Don't worry. I will.

💿 LET'S MASTER THE DIALOGUE!

Now repeat the main dialogue at natural speed with the CD.

💿 LISTENING

A : Listen to the dialogue. Then circle the correct answer for each question.

CDの会話を聞き，それぞれの質問に対する正解を（　　）で囲みなさい。

1. now	soon	much later
2. sluggish	tired	drowsy
3. tiredness	medicine	lack of sleep
4. yes	no	not known
5. very long	not very long	not known

B : Listen to the questions and write your answers on the lines.

CDの質問に対して，自分について答えなさい。

1. _____
2. _____
3. _____
4. _____

UNIT 5 POSTOPERATIVE CARE

DIALOGUE 1 — OBSERVATION AFTER OPERATION (1)

Nurse: Do you feel nauseated?

Patient: Yes, I do.

Nurse: If you have to vomit, please let me know.

Patient: If I don't have time to call you, what do I do?

Nurse: I'll put a kidney basin next to your pillow.

Patient: Thank you.

Nurse: Does your foot hurt?

Patient: No, it doesn't.

Nurse: Can you wiggle your toes?

Patient: Only slightly.

Nurse: It's still numb from the anesthetic. You'll regain full movement soon.

Patient: That's good to hear.

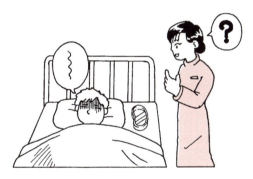

KEY SENTENCES	KEY WORDS AND PHRASES
1. Do you feel nauseated? 2. I'll put a kidney basin next to your pillow. 3. Can you wiggle your toes? 4. You'll regain full movement soon.	nauseated vomit kidney basin numb wiggle toe regain movement

UNIT 5-1

🔘 **EXERCISE 1** —Repeat each sentence in the dialogue after the tape.

🔘 **EXERCISE 2** —Repeat the key sentences.
　　　　　　　 Repeat the key words and phrases.

EXERCISE 3 —Let's learn the key sentences!

N: Do you feel _____ ?

P: _____.

N: That's not good. / That's good.

---

1. nauseated

    Yes, a little

2. sick

    Yes, very much

3. restless

    Yes, I do

4. tired

    Not really

5. sleepy

    Not at all

P: If I don't have time to call you, what do I do?

N: I'll put a _____

　　_____ your _____.

P: Thanks. That makes me feel better.

N: Good.

---

1. kidney basin

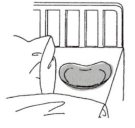

next to
pillow

2. a box of tissue paper

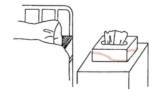

on
night table

3. urinal

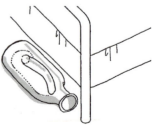

under
bed

UNIT 5-1

N: Can you _____ your _____?
P: _____.
N: That's good. / Don't worry. Soon you can.

1. wiggle / toes

   Yes, I can

2. bend / knees

   Only slightly

3. stretch / arm

   Not very much

4. move / fingers

   No problem

5. twist / neck

   No, I can't

N: You'll regain full _____ soon.
P: How soon?
N: Oh, in _____.

1. movement
   several hours

2. energy
   a week or two

3. strength
   a few weeks

UNIT 5-1

Master the Expressions!

Choose the most suitable word or phrase for each blank from the bottom and complete the conversation.

下記より最も適切な語を選び，空欄を埋め会話を完成させなさい。

N: Do you feel _____ ?

P: Not now.

N: Whenever you do, _____ .

P: Okay, but if I'm really in a hurry, what should I do?

N: I'll put a _____ next _____ your pillow just in case.

P: That's good.

N: Can you _____ your toes?

P: Not very much.

N: Don't worry, you'll _____ full _____ soon.

hungry	a urinal	nauseated	movement	kidney basin
appetite	please let us know	tired	please hurry	wiggle
from	to	at	twist	regain

EXERCISE 4 ― Nausea and Vomit　吐き気と嘔吐

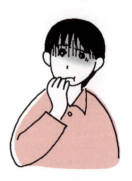

nausea：吐き気

吐き気がする―feel（be）nauseated, have nausea

Do you feel nauseated / sick?

Are you nauseated?

Do you have any nausea?

＊sick は，単に病気という意味以外に以下のような使われ方をするとムカムカするとか，今にも吐きそうという意味になる。

I feel sick (nauseated).　ムカムカする。

I'm going to be sick (vomit).　今にも吐きそう。

UNIT 5-1

vomit：嘔吐

Do you feel like vomiting?

Do you have (need) to vomit?

Have you had any vomiting?

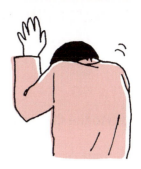

＊vomitの他に一般的に使われる口語表現にthrow upがある。
I vomited up my supper last night. / I threw up my lunch.

吐血する

He vomited some blood this morning.

Have you had any vomiting of blood?

喀血する

Have you coughed up any blood?

Master the Expressions!

Fill each blank with a word so that the top and bottom sentences may have about the same meaning.

a．b．の両方の文がほぼ同じ意味になるように（　　）の中に一語入れなさい。

1. a．I threw up dinner last night.
   b．I（　　　）up dinner last night.
2. a．Are you feeling sick?
   b．Do you feel（　　　）?
3. a．Do you feel you have to vomit?
   b．Do you feel（　　　）（　　　）?
4. a．Have you thrown up any food?
   b．Have you（　　　）any（　　　）?
5. a．Do you have nausea?
   b．（　　　）you（　　　）?

UNIT 5-1

💿 LET'S MASTER THE DIALOGUE!

Now repeat the main dialogue at natural speed with the CD.

💿 LISTENING

Listen to the CD and write True or False.

CDの内容に合っているものにはT（true）を，合っていないものにはF（false）を（　）の中に記入しなさい。

(　) 1. The patient is feeling sick.

(　) 2. The patient has to vomit.

(　) 3. The nurse will bring a kidney basin later.

(　) 4. The patient had an operation on her leg.

(　) 5. The patient is feeling the pain now.

(　) 6. The patient is still under the influence of the anesthetic.

(　) 7. The patient can wiggle her toes very well.

(　) 8. The patient will get full movement back in two or three hours.

UNIT 5-2

DIALOGUE 2 —OBSERVATION AFTER OPERATION (2)

Nurse: (Checking a thermometer:) You have a fever. Do you have a headache?

Patient: No, I don't.

Nurse: Your forehead feels hot. Would you like an ice bag?

Patient: No, that's not necessary right now.

Nurse: Well, then just press this call button when you need any help.

Patient: Okay.

Nurse: When this bottle is empty, it'll be replaced with another IV bottle.

Patient: Another one?

Nurse: Yes. You can't eat or drink anything until the anesthetic wears off.

Patient: I see. Can I gargle if my mouth gets dry?

Nurse: Sure.

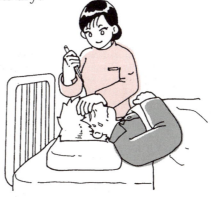

KEY SENTENCES

1. Would you like an ice bag?
2. Just press this call button when you need any help.
3. When this bottle is empty, it'll be replaced with another IV bottle.
4. You can't eat or drink anything until the anesthetic wears off.

KEY WORDS AND PHRASES

forehead
ice bag
call button
empty
eat and drink
until
wear off
sure

〔ノート〕
ここではIV bottleという表現を使用しているが，特殊な輸液を除いては，現在は点滴にはボトルよりバッグを使用する場合が多いので，IV bagという表現の方が一般的である。

UNIT 5-2

🔴 **EXERCISE 1** —Repeat each sentence in the dialogue after the CD.

🔴 **EXERCISE 2** —Repeat the key sentences.
　　　　　　　Repeat the key words and phrases.

EXERCISE 3 —Let's learn the key sentences!

　　　　　＿＿＿上にはKEY SENTENCESで学んだ単語を思い出して入れて練習してください。

N: Would you like ＿＿＿＿＿＿＿＿＿＿＿＿＿＿＿＿＿?

P: Yes, that'd be nice.

N: Okay, I'll bring it/them right now.

P: Thank you.

---

1. an ice bag　　　2. some magazines　　　3. some water

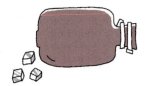 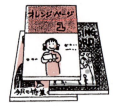 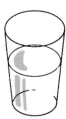

N: Just ＿＿＿＿ this call button when you ＿＿＿＿＿＿＿＿＿＿＿＿.

P: Okay.

N: I'll check back in a few minutes.

---

1. don't feel well　　2. would like to use the bathroom　　3. need any help

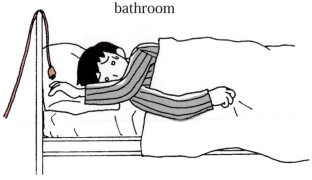

UNIT 5-2

N: When this _____ is _____ , it'll be _____ with
_____ .

P: Then I don't need to worry.

N: Right. We'll take care of it.

P: Great.

1. bag/full/a new bag   2. IV bag/empty/another   3. ice bag / warm / a fresh one

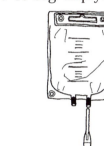
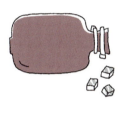
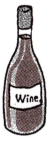

N: You can't _____ until _____ .

P: No _____ ?

N: That's right. Please bear with it.

P: I'll try.

1. have any alcoholic drinks

   the test results come back

2. eat or drink

   the anesthetic wears off

3. take a bath

   the wound heals

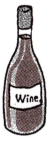
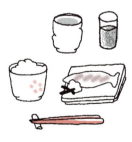
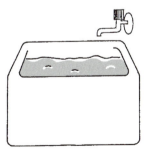

alcohol   food or drink   bath

UNIT 5-2

Master the Expressions!

Complete the conversation by filling each blank with one word.

各空欄に一語ずつ入れて会話を完成させなさい。

N: How are you _____?

P: I'm all right.

N: _____ you _____ something to read?

P: No, thank you.

N: _____ this IV bottle _____ empty, it will _____ _____ with another one.

P: One more?

N: Right. Because you can't have anything _____ the anesthetic wears off.

P: I see.

N: Well, if you need any assistance, just _____ this _____ button.

P: Okay I will.

EXERCISE 4 —Feel, Taste, Look, and Sound   感覚動詞の使い方を覚えよう。

Read each set of sentences and discuss the difference in connotation.

それぞれ二つの文を読んでその意味の違いを話し合いなさい。

1. It feels very soft.

   It is very soft.

2. It tastes good.

   It is good.

3. That house looks great.

   That house is great.

4. The plan sounds nice.

   The plan is nice.

UNIT 5-2

Master the Expressions!

Fill in each blank with either feel, taste, look, or sound.
feel, taste, look, soundのいずれかを各空欄に記入しなさい。語形は主語に応じて変更のこと。

1. A：I'm going to go to Europe this summer.
   B：Oh, that _____ great.
2. A：Would you like to try this salad?
   B：Sure.（After trying：）Oh, this _____ delicious.
3. A：It's really cold, isn't it?
   B：Yeah, my hands _____ so cold.
4. A：How do you like this new dress of mine?
   B：Oh, you _____ wonderful!

LET'S MASTER THE DIALOGUE!
Now repeat the main dialogue at natural speed with the CD.

LISTENING
Listen to the dialogue. Then answer the following questions.
CDの対話を聞き，以下の質問に答えなさい。

1. Where should the patient place the thermometer?
   _____.
2. How long does he have to keep it there?
   _____.
3. What is the temperature of the patient in Fahrenheit?
   _____.
4. Does the patient want an ice bag?
   _____.
5. What does he have to do if he needs any help?
   _____.
6. Is the patient going to get another IV bottle?
   _____.
7. How long does the patient have to wait before he starts eating again?
   _____.

UNIT 5-3

DIALOGUE 3 —URINARY CATHETERIZATION (1)

Nurse: How may I help you?

Patient: I have to urinate.

Nurse: I'll bring you a urinal.

　　　(The nurse returns with a urinal.)

Nurse: Just press the call button when you're finished.

Patient: All right, I will.

　　　(The patient presses the call button.)

Nurse: Are you finished?

Patient: No. My bladder feels full, but I can't pass any urine.

Nurse: Your bladder does seem full.

Patient: It hurts so much. Could you please help me?

Nurse: It's best if you can urinate without using a catheter.

Patient: But I can't.

Nurse: Why don't I massage your lower abdomen a little bit?

Patient: (Receiving massage:) It hurts, it hurts.

KEY SENTENCES

1. How may I help you?
2. Your bladder seems full.
3. It's best if you can urinate without using a catheter.
4. Why don't I massage your abdomen?

KEY WORDS AND PHRASES

urinary catheterization
urinate
urinal
bladder
pass urine
catheter
massage
abdomen

〔ノート〕
導尿用に使われるカテーテル（留置カテーテル）は，英語ではFoley catheterと呼ばれる。ただし，専門用語なので患者に対しては使わない。

UNIT 5-3

EXERCISE 1 —Repeat each sentence in the dialogue after the CD.

EXERCISE 2 —Repeat the key sentences.
　　　　　　　Repeat the key words and phrases.

EXERCISE 3 —Let's learn the key sentences!

　　　　------ 上にはKEY SENTENCESで学んだ単語を思い出して入れて練習してください。

（A nurse hears a call button buzzing and comes to the patient's room.）

N : _____ I _____ you?

P : Would you raise my head a little bit?

N : Sure.

1．How may　　　　　2．What can　　　　　3．How can

　　help　　　　　　　　do for　　　　　　　　help

P : My lower abdomen feels very uncomfortable.

N : Your bladder ------------------------.

　　Do you have pain?

P : Yes, it hurts. Can you do something about it?

N : I'll see what I can do.

1．full　　　　　　　2．distended　　　　　3．filled

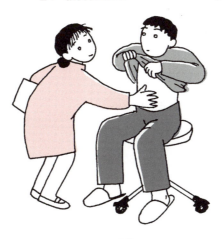

UNIT 5-3

P: I'm having trouble _____.
　　Can you give me something that'll help?
N: It's best if you can _____ -------------- _____.
P: All right. I'll try.

1. passing urine
　　urinate
　　using a catheter

2. falling asleep
　　sleep
　　any medication

3. passing stools
　　excrete
　　taking a laxative

P: My back is sore.
N: _____ massage your back?
P: That'd be great.

1. Why don't I
2. Would you like me to
3. Shall I

Master the Expressions!

Fill in each space with a correct word.

空欄を適切な単語で埋めなさい。

N: _____ _____ I help you?

P: My shoulders are really stiff.

N: Let's see. Yes, your neck and shoulders _____ very tight.

P: Can you give me some medication?

N: I can ask your doctor, but it's _____ _____ you can relax your muscles _____ taking any medication.

P: But how?

N: _____ _____ I show you some exercises that will help?

P: That'd be very helpful. I'll try.

EXERCISE 4 — It does seem full. 強調

Learn the intonation of sentences with stressed words by practicing out loud with a partner.

強勢のある文のイントネーションを，パートナーと組になって声に出して練習してみよう。

Regular verbs　一般動詞の場合：

1．P: I have a pain in my abdomen.　　　N: Your bladder *does* seem full.
2．P: I feel great today.　　　　　　　　N: You *do* look good.
3．P: I had a good night's sleep.
　　　I slept for nine hours last night.　　N: You *did* sleep very well.

Auxiliary verbs and be-verbs　助動詞，be 動詞の場合：

1．P: I can't do it.　　　　　　　　　　　N: Yes, you *can*.
2．P: How am I doing? Am I getting better?　N: Yes, you *are*.
3．P: My bladder was full, wasn't it?　　　N: Yes, it *was*.
4．P: I have been working hard.　　　　　N: You sure *have*.

Master the Expressions!

Fill in each blank with a word to stress the following verb.

空欄の次の動詞を強調するように空欄を埋めて文を完成させなさい。

1．P: I think I have a fever. I don't feel very well.
　　N: You _____ have a fever.
2．P: There is something wrong with my neck. I can't move it.
　　N: Your neck _____ feel stiff.
3．P: I took a long walk yesterday. I walked a mile.
　　N: You _____ take a long walk. Good for you!

UNIT 5-3

🔴 LET'S MASTER THE DIALOGUE!

Now repeat the main dialogue at natural speed with the CD.

🔴 LISTENING

Listen to each dialogue and write the most stressed word in the nurse's part.

会話を聞き，看護師のセンテンスの中で最も強調されていることばを書き出しなさい。

1. _____
2. _____
3. _____
4. _____
5. _____

DIALOGUE 4 —URINARY CATHETERIZATION (2)

Nurse: Let me go and get a catheter. I'll be back in a few minutes.

Patient: Please hurry.

Nurse: (Returns quickly:) Inserting the catheter may be slightly painful, so please bear with me.

Patient: I'll try.

Nurse: (The catheter is inserted.) The catheter will draw off the urine from your bladder now. Try to relax and breathe naturally.

Patient: All right.

Nurse: It seems to be working. (A few minutes later:) Your bladder *was* distended. It must have been very painful for you.

Patient: It certainly was.

Nurse: How do you feel now?

Patient: Much better. Thank you so much.

Nurse: You're welcome.

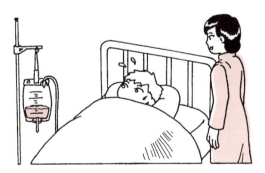

KEY SENTENCES	KEY WORDS AND PHRASES
1. I'll be back in a few minutes.	insert
2. Inserting the catheter may be slightly painful.	draw off
3. Try to relax.	breathe
4. You're welcome.	naturally
	distended

UNIT 5-4

🔴 **EXERCISE 1** ―Repeat each sentence in the dialogue after the CD.

🔴 **EXERCISE 2** ―Repeat the key sentences.
　　　　　　　Repeat the key words and phrases.

EXERCISE 3 ―Let's learn the key sentences!

　　　　　上にはKEY SENTENCESで学んだ単語を思い出して入れて練習してください。

> N: How may I help you?*
> P: I'd like _____ .
> N: Okay. I'll go and get _____ . I'll be back _____ .

*Or: What can I do for you?

1. a pen and a sheet of paper

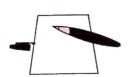

them / shortly

2. another blanket

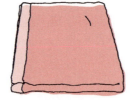

one / in a few minutes

3. some water

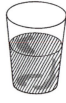

some / soon

> N: _____ may be slightly painful.
> P: Try to be as gentle as possible.
> N: I'll try my best.

1. Disinfecting the wound

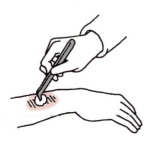

2. Inserting the catheter

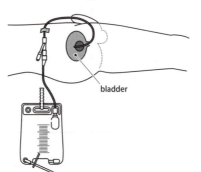

3. Removing the gauze

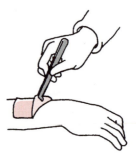

UNIT 5-4

N: We are going to start the test.

P: Oh, I'm nervous.

N: Don't be nervous. Try _____.

P: I'll try.

1．to ease your mind   2．not to worry too much   3．to relax

N: How do you _____ now?

P: Oh, I feel much better. Thank you so much.

N: _____. I'm glad you're feeling better.

1．You're welcome.   2．My pleasure.   3．Don't mention it.
4．It's my pleasure.   5．You bet.

Master the Expressions!

Fill in the blanks. The word should start with the given letter on the line.

空欄を埋めなさい。各語は空欄上の文字で始まる。

1．Please don't be so nervous. Try to r_____.

2．I won't be so late. I'll be b_____ in a few hours.

3．I_____ the catheter may be painful.

4．N: The catheter will d_____ o_____ your urine now.

　　P: Thank you.

　　N: Y_____ w_____.

5．Try to b_____ naturally.

6．N: Your bladder seems to be d_____. It must be uncomfortable.

　　P: It's very p_____.

UNIT 5-4

EXERCISE 4 —It must have been very painful.

助動詞＋完了形（have＋過去分詞）：仮定法

must (mustn't) have＋past participle	〜したにちがいない（〜すべきではなかった）
should (shouldn't) have＋past participle	〜すべきだった（〜すべきではなかった）
would (wouldn't) have＋past participle	〜しただろう（〜しなかっただろう）
could (couldn't) have＋past participle	〜することができたはずだ（〜することは到底できなかっただろう／したはずがない）
might (might not) have＋past participle	〜したかもしれない（しなかったかもしれない）

Examples:

You must have forgotten about me.

You should have told me about your pain.

I would have done the same.

I could have helped you better.

I might have put it there.

Master the Expressions!

Choose the most suitable word for each blank to complete the dialogue.

下記よりも最も適切な語を下記より選び，対話を完成させなさい。

P: I think I have a fever. I don't feel very well.

W: You _____ have _____ in bed.

P: My stomach hurts. I have diarrhea.

W: You _____ have _____ something wrong for dinner.

P: The nurse might have given me a wrong medicine.

W: Oh, no. She _____ have _____ such a mistake.

---

a. must　　b. should　　c. would　　d. could　　e. might　　f. mustn't

g. shouldn't　　h. wouldn't　　i. couldn't　　j. done　　k. kept　　l. made

m. eaten　　n. left　　o. given　　p. stayed

UNIT 5-4

💿 LET'S MASTER THE DIALOGUE!
Now repeat the main dialogue at natural speed with the CD.

💿 LISTENING
Listen to each dialogue and circle a. or b. for the correct answer.
CDの会話を聞き，a．b．いずれか内容に合った方を○で囲みなさい。

1. a. The nurse is sure that the patient had great pain.
   b. The nurse is not sure if the patient had pain or not.
2. a. The nurse thinks the patient made a stupid mistake.
   b. The nurse doesn't think the patient made a stupid mistake.
3. a. The nurse is sure what she was doing when her former patient stopped by at the Nurses' Station.
   b. The nurse is not sure what she was doing when her former patient stopped by at the Nurses' Station.
4. a. The nurse's vacation was very good.
   b. The nurse's vacation wasn't very good.
5. a. The nurse came to help the patient much earlier than expected.
   b. The nurse didn't come to help the patient soon.

UNIT 6 PATIENT DISCHARGE

DIALOGUE 1 —INSTRUCTIONS BEFORE DISCHARGE

Nurse: Congratulations! It's time for your discharge, Mr. Ordal.

Patient: Thank you. I really appreciate everyone's care and helpfulness.

Nurse: Since your wife is here, let's talk about the care after your discharge.

Patient: All right.

Nurse: For a while you'll have some difficulty walking because your right foot is still tender.

Patient: I understand.

Nurse: You'll probably try to favor that foot and walk with a slight limp.

Patient: Is there anything particular to watch out for?

Nurse: Be very careful not to stumble, and take extra care on the stairs.

Patient: Okay I will. What kind of exercise should I do for rehabilitation?

Nurse: When you take a bath, relax your whole body. Then bend and stretch your ankle in the warm water.

Patient: That sounds like a good exercise. Thanks for your advice.

KEY SENTENCES

1. Let's talk about the care after your discharge.
2. You'll probably try to favor that foot.
3. Be very careful not to stumble.

KEY WORDS AND PHRASES

discharge
congratulations
tender
limp
watch out for
take extra care
rehabilitation
take a bath

UNIT 6-1

EXERCISE 1 ─ Repeat each sentence in the dialogue after the tape.

EXERCISE 2 ─ Repeat the key sentences.
　　　　　　　　Repeat the key words and phrases.

EXERCISE 3 ─ Let's learn the key sentences!

　　　　　上にはKEY SENTENCESで学んだ単語を思い出して入れて練習してください。

> N: Let's _____ about _____ after your discharge.
> P: All right.
> N: First, I have to ask you to follow my instructions strictly.
> P: I understand.

1. the medication　　2. the diet　　3. the care

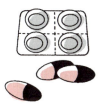 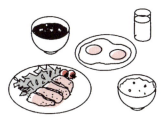 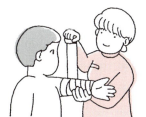

> N: You'll have some difficulty walking for a while.
> P: Why?
> N: Since your _____ is still tender, you'll probably try to favor it.
> P: That's true.

1. right foot　　2. left knee　　3. right ankle

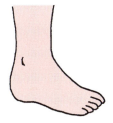 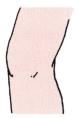 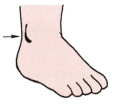

UNIT 6-1

> P: My toe still feels tender when I walk.
> N: Be very _____ not to _____ .
> P: I'll try not to.

1. stub it　　　　2. trip over　　　　3. stumble

Master the Expressions!

Rewrite the following sentences by replacing the underlined words or phrases with other word(s). Keep the meanings the same.

下線部を他の単語や語句に置き替えて文を書き直しなさい。ただし，文意は変えないこと。

1. <u>Why don't we</u> discuss your rehabilitation plan?

2. <u>Take extra care</u> not to fall down.

3. Since your knee is still sore, you'll try to <u>protect</u> it when you walk.

4. What kind of things do I have to <u>be careful about</u>?

EXERCISE 4 —Rehabilitation

リハビリテーション分野の職種と役割を英語で覚えよう。

1. Physical therapy—physical therapist
   The therapy in this field helps people who have difficulty using major muscles, such as people having difficulty walking.

2. Speech pathology (therapy)—speech pathologist (therapist)
   The therapy in this field helps people who have difficulty speaking, swallowing, hearing, and with memory.

3. Occupational therapy—occupational therapist
   The therapy in this field helps people who have difficulty using small muscles that are needed for daily living skills such as writing, using silverware, and dressing.

4．Recreational therapy—recreational therapist

The therapy in this field helps patients regain old hobbies and pleasure activities, and also develop new pleasure activity skills.

Master the Expressions!

Fill in the blanks in relation to rehabilitation.

リハビリテーションについて空欄に語句を記入しなさい。

1．P: After my operation, I still have difficulty bending my knee.

   N: You may need some _____ _____. I'll let your doctor know.

2．Mr. Smith has difficulty using forks, spoons, and knives when he eats.

   He definitely needs _____ _____.

3．When you are recovering from a long illness, _____ _____ may be helpful to bring you some pleasure in life.

4．After his stroke, Mr. Wright has difficulty speaking and remembering things.

   He is now in therapy with a _____ _____.

🔴 LET'S MASTER THE DIALOGUE!

Now repeat the main dialogue at natural speed with the CD.

🔴 LISTENING

Listen to the CD and write each person's problem and the recommended care. If there is none, put an × in the box.

CDを聞き，それぞれの患者の状態（問題）とそれに対するケアを聴きとり，空欄に記入しなさい。もし，あてはまるものがなければ×を記入しなさい。

	PROBLEM	RECOMMENDED CARE
1．Mr. Stevens		
2．Ms. Taylor		
3．Mrs. Andrews		
4．Miss Jordan		

UNIT 6-2

DIALOGUE 2 —INSTRUCTION ON DIET

Nurse: Since your blood pressure is sometimes high, you should reduce the amount of salt in your diet. Low-salt diets are good for health.

Patient's Wife: The hospital nutritionist gave me some advice for preparing low-salt meals.

Nurse: Good. I also recommend low-fat meals.

Patient's Wife: That's a good idea. By the way, are *miso* soup and *nattō* frequently served here also recommended for my husband's diet?

Nurse: They are very good for health, but start with the foods you like. Just don't forget to reduce your salt intake.

Patient: I'm relieved to learn that I don't have to eat *nattō*. If you said yes, my wife would serve it every day.

Patient's Wife: I'll try my best to prepare low-salt and low-fat meals. Thank you very much for your advice. You have been most informative.

Nurse: You're very welcome.

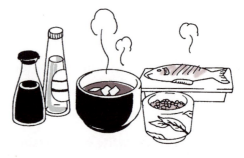

KEY SENTENCES

1. You should reduce the amount of salt in your diet.
2. Low-salt diets are good for health.
3. Start with the foods you like.
4. Don't forget to reduce your salt intake.

KEY WORDS AND PHRASES

diet
the amount of salt
low-salt
low-fat
frequently
be recommended for
salt intake
be relieved

UNIT **6**-2

💿 **EXERCISE 1**—Repeat each sentence in the dialogue after the CD.

💿 **EXERCISE 2**—Repeat the key sentences.
　　　　　　　Repeat the key words and phrases.

EXERCISE 3—Let's learn the key sentences!

　　　_ _ _ _ _ 上にはKEY SENTENCESで学んだ単語を思い出して入れて練習してください。

> P: What should I watch out for in my diet?
> N: You should _____ _____ _____.
> P: Oh, that's tough. I love _____.
> N: I know, but it's very important for your health.
> P: Okay. I'll try my best.

1. sugar　　　　　2. salt　　　　　3. fat

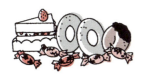　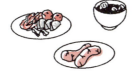　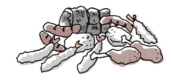

　　sweet stuff　　　　　salty food　　　　　fried food

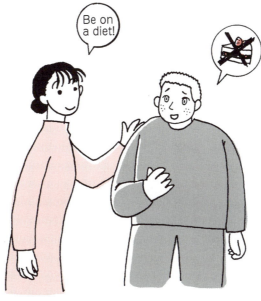

UNIT 6-2

P: The hospital dietitian* told me to _____ the amount of _____ in my diet.

N: _____ are very good for health.

P: I know, but it takes a great effort.

N: Yes, but it'll pay off** in the long run.

*nutritionist   **be worthwhile

1. increase / vegetables   2. cut down / salt   3. reduce / fat

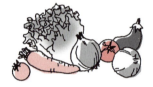 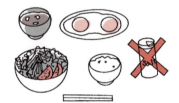 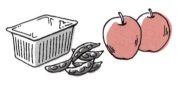

Vegetables   Low-salt diets   Low-fat foods

N: You have to pay attention to getting more exercise.

P: Do I need to belong to an athletic club?

N: No, you don't have to. _____ with _____ you _____.

P: I like that idea.

1. the exercise /   2. light exercise /   3. anything /
   like   can handle   feel comfortable with

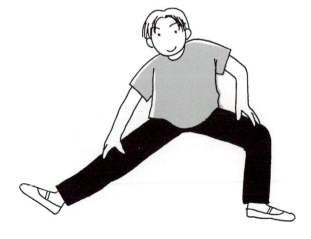

—108—

UNIT 6-2

> N: Congratulations on your recovery!
>
> P: Thank you very much. I feel great.
>
> N: That's good, but don't forget to _____.
>
> P: Don't worry. I won't.

1. get enough sleep   2. reduce your salt intake   3. take medicine

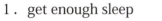
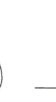
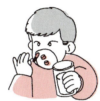

Master the Expressions!

Fill in each blank with a suitable word to complete the conversation between a patient and a nurse.

各空欄に一語を入れ，下記の看護師と患者の会話を完成させなさい。

N: Have you talked with one of the nutritionists about your _____ at home yet?

P: Yes, I have. She told me that I should _____ the amount of _____ in my _____ for my high blood pressure.
　She also recommended _____ meals by cutting some of the greasy foods I have been eating. She said it's best for my health.

N: Did she give you some advice for _____ those meals?

P: Yes, my wife got full instructions. I hope she won't overdo it.

W: Don't worry. The nutritionist said that my husband can _____ with the _____ he likes. I will be careful about the amount of salt and fat when preparing meals.

N: Oh, that's good.

P: I wonder if I can enjoy my meals.

N: I'm sure your wife will prepare wonderful meals. Relax and enjoy your meals. Just don't _____ to _____ your salt and fat _____ _____ _____.

UNIT 6-2

EXERCISE 4 —Adverbs of Frequency 頻度を表すいろいろな副詞

```
0%            25%          50%          75%          100%
|-------------|------------|------------|------------|
never        sometimes    often        frequently   always
almost never occasionally              almost always
seldom       once in a while  very often   very frequently
rarely
```

※数字と副詞は必ずしも完全に一致するわけではなく，あくまでもだいたいの目安として考える。何の頻度について話しているかにより（例えば，普通毎日するものか，普通月に1回程度のものか等），同じ副詞でもその表す頻度は変化してくる。

EXAMPLES：

I never fail to check my patients' charts in the morning.

Mr. Harris sometimes does the laundry by himself.

I rarely eat lunch outside the hospital.

Master the Expressions!

Looking at the chart above, rewrite the following sentences using the adverbs of frequency listed above.

下記のそれぞれの文章で表している頻度は，どのような副詞で置き替えられるか考え，その副詞を使って文を書き替えなさい。

1．I have to work on the night shift about half of the week.
2．I never forget to return calls.
3．I eat dinner out about once a week.
4．Mr. Wiss does not watch TV at all.
5．I study English at home five days a week.

UNIT **6**-2

🔴 LET'S MASTER THE DIALOGUE!
Now repeat the main dialogue at natural speed with the CD.

🔴 LISTENING
Listen to the dialogue, then listen to the questions and circle the right answers.
You can circle more than one.

会話の内容を聞きとり，各質問に対する正解を○で囲みなさい。正解は一つ以上の場合もある。

1. a．overwork   b．overweight   c．loss of weight

2. a．chicken   b．fried food   c．pork

3. a．swimming   b．jogging   c．walking

4. a．a total change   b．a moderate change   c．a very small change
      in diet   in diet   in diet

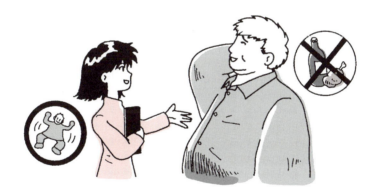

UNIT 6-3

DIALOGUE 3 —APPOINTMENT AS AN OUTPATIENT

Head Nurse: Mr. Ordal, you've made a speedy recovery.

Patient: Thanks to your care.

Nurse: Please return to the Outpatient Clinic two weeks from today on Wednesday.

Patient: At what time?

Nurse: Your appointment is scheduled for 10:00 o'clock in the morning.

Patient: What's the date?

Nurse: It's November 5.

Patient: At 10:00 o'clock on November 5. Okay.

Nurse: Please go to the Outpatient Reception Desk before 10:00 o'clock. Then give your hospital ID card and appointment card to the receptionist.

Patient: Do I need to bring my health insurance booklet too?

Nurse: No. Go to Outpatient Orthopedics and wait in the waiting room.

Patient: Will Doctor Higuchi examine me?

Nurse: Yes, he will. Have you completed the discharge paperwork and paid the hospital bill?

Patient's Wife: Yes. I've just finished everything with Accounting.

Nurse: Good. If you have any trouble at home, please don't hesitate to phone us.

Patient and his wife:

Thank you very much for everything.

Nurse and Head Nurse:

Take good care of yourself.

UNIT 6-3

KEY SENTENCES

1. You've made a speedy recovery.
2. Your appointment is scheduled for 10:00 o'clock in the morning.
3. Have you completed the discharge paperwork?
4. Please don't hesitate to phone us.

KEY WORDS AND PHRASES

outpatient
outpatient clinic
appointment
be scheduled for
hospital ID card
Outpatient Orthopedics
waiting room
appointment card
discharge paperwork
hospital bill
take care of

EXERCISE 1 —Repeat each sentence in the dialogue after the CD.

EXERCISE 2 —Repeat the key sentences.
　　　　　　　Repeat the key words and phrases.

EXERCISE 3 —Let's learn the key sentences!

　　　　　　上にはKEY SENTENCESで学んだ単語を思い出して入れて練習してください。

N: You will be discharged the day after tomorrow.

P: The day after tomorrow. That's great.

N: You've made a ＿＿＿＿＿＿＿＿＿＿＿.

P: Thanks to your care.

---

1. speedy　　　　2. nice　　　　3. quick

N: I've made an appointment for your first outpatient visit.

P: When is that?

N: Your appointment is scheduled ＿＿＿＿＿＿＿ next ＿＿＿＿＿.

P: All right.

---

1. 9:30 a.m.　　　　2. 2:00 p.m.　　　　3. 10:00 a.m.
　 Thursday　　　　　 Tuesday　　　　　　 Monday

UNIT 6-3

> N: Have you _____ the _____ ?
> P: Yes, I have.
> N: Good. You're all set to leave the hospital.
> P: Great.

1. paid / hospital bill　　2. completed / discharge paperwork　　3. filled out / form

> N: Please don't hesitate to _____ us anytime if you have _____ .
> P: Thanks.
> N: Then please _____ good care of yourself.
> P: I will. Good-by.

1. call / any trouble　　2. phone / a question　　3. contact / a problem

Master the Expressions!

Fill in each blank with a suitable word to complete the conversation between a patient and a nurse.

下記の看護師と患者の会話の内容をよく把握しながら，各空欄に一語を入れ，会話を完成させなさい。

N: Miss Foley, you've _____ a speedy _____ .

P: Yes, _____ to your excellent care.

N: I've just made an _____ for your first visit as an _____ .

P: Oh, thank you. When is it?

N: It is _____ for 11:00 in the morning on November 10.

P: Okay, let me write it down so that I may not forget.

N: Have you completed the _____ paperwork?

P: Yes, I've finished everything.

N: Good. Well, take care, and don't _____ to phone us if you have any _____ at home.

UNIT 6-3

EXERCISE 4 —Days, Dates, and Specifying a day or a date　曜日，日付，日の特定

1. **What day of the week is it today?**　今日は何曜日ですか。

   Read the days of the week out loud.　声を出して読んでみよう。

   | Sunday | Monday | Tuesday | Wednesday |
   | Thursday | Friday | Saturday | |

   Work in a pair and practice asking for a day and giving the answer.

   ペアになって，曜日をたずねる質問と応答の練習をしなさい。

   Q：_____?

   A：_____.

2. **What's the date today?**　今日は何日ですか。

   Read the months of the year out loud.

   | January | February | March | April | May | June | July |
   | August | September | October | November | December | | |

   Read the dates out loud.

1 ＝ first	2 ＝ second	3 ＝ third
4 ＝ forth	5 ＝ fifth	6 ＝ sixth
7 ＝ seventh	8 ＝ eighth	9 ＝ ninth
10 ＝ tenth	11 ＝ eleventh	12 ＝ twelfth
13 ＝ thirteenth	14 ＝ fourteenth	15 ＝ fifteenth
20 ＝ twentieth	30 ＝ thirtieth	31 ＝ thirty-first

   Read the following.

   A：What's the date today?

   B：It's December 23（twenty-third）

   Work in a pair and practice asking for a date and giving the answer.

   ペアになって日付の聞き方，答え方の練習をしなさい。

   Q：_____?

   A：_____.

UNIT 6-3

3. **When?**—Let's learn various expressions for a specific time.

   日を特定するいろいろな表現を学ぼう。

   Future 未来：

   tomorrow   the day after tomorrow   this Friday   this weekend

   next Friday   a week from today   the week after next

   a month from now   the month after next   a year from now

   the year after next

   Past 過去：

   yesterday   the day before yesterday   last Friday   last weekend

   Friday before last   a week ago   a month ago   a year ago

   the week before last   the month before last   the year before last

Use a calendar and practice asking specific days and dates and giving the answers.

下の例にならい，カレンダーを使って，特定の曜日や日付のたずね方，答え方を練習してみよう。

EXAMPLES：

   Q: When did you see him?

   A: It was Sunday before last.

   Q: December 5?

   A: That's right.

Master the Expressions!

▮ is today's date. Looking at the calendar, answer the questions below.

▮ 今日の日付である。カレンダーを見て，下記の質問に答えなさい。

JANUARY

SUN	MON	TUE	WED	THU	FRI	SAT
1	2	3	4	5	6	7
8	9	10	11	12	13	14
15	16	17	18	19	20	21
22	23	24	25	26	27	28
29	30	31				

UNIT 6-3

1. What is the date today?
2. What day of the week is it?
3. What day is January 20?
4. What's the date two weeks from today?
5. What's the date a week before last Friday?

LET'S MASTER THE DIALOGUE!

Now repeat the main dialogue at natural speed with the CD.

LISTENING

NOVEMBER

SUN	MON	TUE	WED	THU	FRI	SAT
1	2	3	4	5	6	7
8	9	10	11	12	13	14
15	16	17	18	19	20	21
22	23	24	25	26	27	28
29	30					

Today is November 3.

Listen to the CD as you look at the calendar. Then circle a. b. or c. for the correct information for the next appointment.

カレンダーを見ながらCDを聞きなさい。次回の予約日について正解をそれぞれa～cの中より選び○で囲みなさい。

1. a. 9:00　　Monday, November 9
   b. 11:00　Tuesday, November 10
   c. 11:00　Monday, November 9

2. a. 9:00　　Wednesday, November 4
   b. 9:30　　Wednesday, November 18
   c. 9:00　　Wednesday, November 25

3. a. 2:00　　Friday, November 13
   b. 2:00　　Monday, November 16
   c. 2:00　　Friday, November 20

Parts of a human body

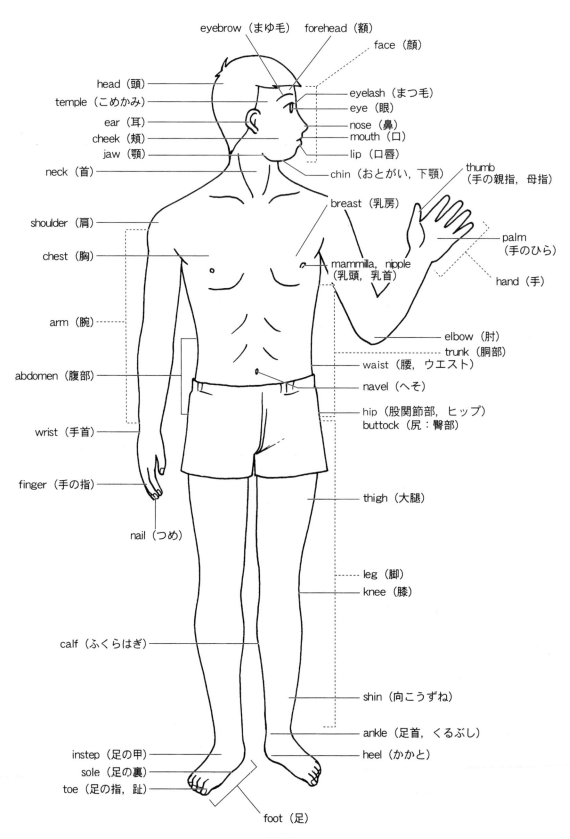

Human organs

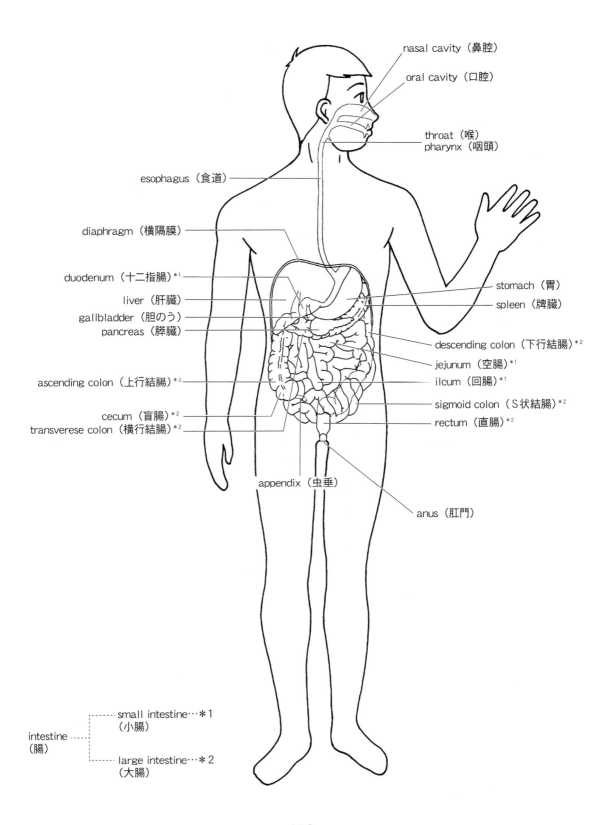

Human organs

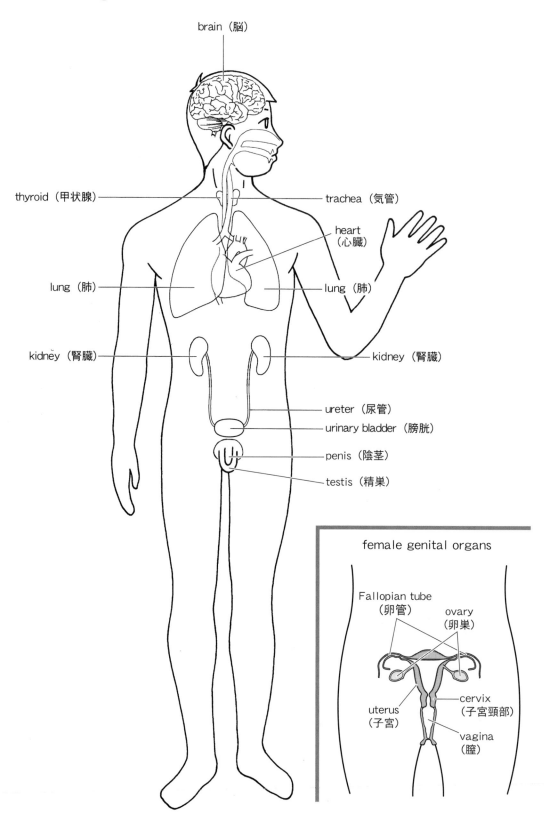

Skeleton

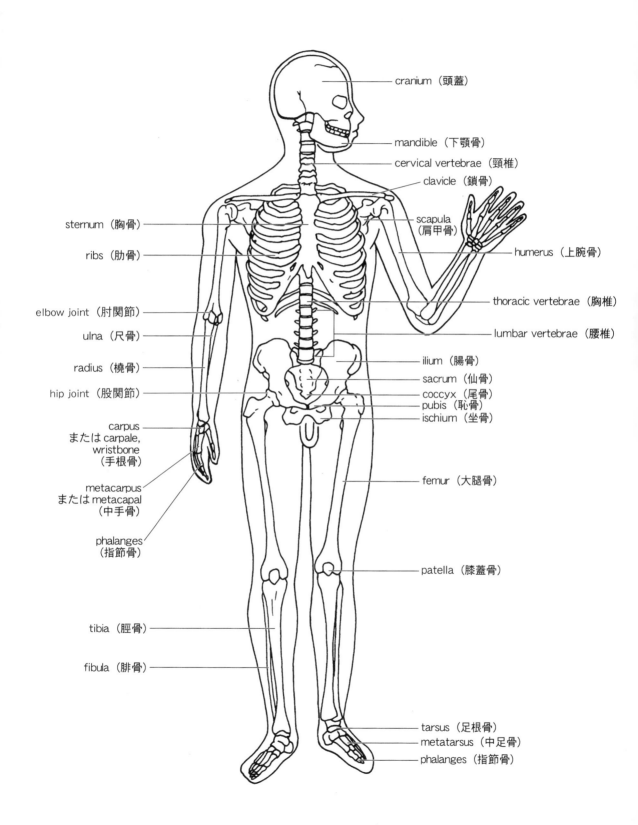

List of Professionals and Departments in Hospital
診療科や医療職などに関する単語

職種，役職，立場などの名称

医師	physician / medical doctor（MD）
歯科医師	dentist
薬剤師	pharmacist
理学療法士	physical therapist（PT）
作業療法士	occupational therapist（OT）
言語聴覚士	speech pathologist／therapist（ST）
レクリエーション療法士	recreational therapist
医療ソーシャルワーカー	(medical) social worker（MSW）
栄養士	dietitian（dietician）／nutritionist
管理栄養士	registered dietitian
放射線技師	radiology technologist, radiology technician
臨床検査技師	medical technician
救命救急士	paramedic
助産師	nurse-midwife
専門看護師	clinical nurse specialist
認定看護師	certified _____ nurse（専門科名，例 oncology）
診療看護師	nurse practitioner
正看護師	registered nurse（RN）
准看護師	licensed practical nurse（LPN）／vocational technical nurse（VTN）
認定看護助手	certified nursing assistant（CNA）
看護補助者	nurse's aide
病棟事務職員	unit secretary
医師事務作業補助者	medical clerk

電話交換手	(telephone) operator
警備員	guard, security person

内科医	medical internist, a specialist in internal medicine
外科医	surgeon
小児科医	pediatrician
産科医	obstetrician
婦人科医	gynecologist
整形外科医	orthopedist
皮膚科医	dermatologist
泌尿器科医	urologist
眼科医	ophthalmologist
耳鼻咽喉科医	otorhinolaryngologist, otolaryngologist, ENT specialist
放射線科医	radiologist
麻酔科医	anesthesiologist
精神科医	psychiatrist
神経科医	neurologist
脳神経外科医	neurosurgeon
循環器内科医	cardiologist
心臓外科医	cardiothoracic surgeon, cardiac surgeon
呼吸器内科医	pulmonologist
消化器内科医	gastroenterologist
内分泌内科医	endocrinologist
がん専門医	oncologist
リハビリテーション医	physiatrist

院長	chief executive officer（CEO）
副院長	chief operating officer（COO）, vice president
看護部長	director of nursing (service)
副看護部長	assistant director of nursing (service)
師長	nurse manager
主任看護師	assistant nurse manager (charge nurse)
事務長	chief office administrator
教授	professor
准教授	associate professor
講師	lecturer (assistant professor)
医学生	medical student
看護学生	nursing student
1年生	freshman, first-year student
2年生	sophomore, second-year student
3年生	junior, third-year student
4年生	senior, fourth-year student

患者	patient
外来患者	outpatient
入院患者	inpatient
見舞い客	visitor

診療科の名称

内科	internal medicine
外科	surgery
小児科	pediatrics
産科	obstetrics
婦人科	gynecology
整形外科	orthopedics
皮膚科	dermatology
泌尿器科	urology
眼科	ophthalmology
耳鼻咽喉科	ear, nose, and throat (ENT), otorhinolaryngology
放射線科	radiology
麻酔科	anesthesiology
精神科	psychiatry
神経科	neurology
脳神経外科	neurosurgery
心理療法科	psychotherapy
歯科	dentistry
循環器内科	cardiovascular medicine
心臓内科	cardiology
消化器内科	gastroenterology
内分泌科	endocrinology
腫瘍科	oncology
血液内科	hematology
心臓外科	cardiac surgery
胸部心臓外科	cardiothoracic surgery
呼吸器内科	pulmonology
女性専門科	women's health
男性専門科	men's health
リハビリ科	rehabilitation medicine

> **＊診療科の表記について**
>
> 正式な学術論文などにおいてはthe Department of ～（例：the Department of Internal Medicine）であるが，一般に使う場合，病院内，専門職間においてもthe ～ Department（例：the Internal Medicine Department）でよく，さらに簡単にtheもdepartmentもつけずに診療科名だけでもよい．書き表す場合は，それぞれの単語の最初を大文字にする．（例：Internal Medicine）

病院内の施設，部署の名称

科，部	department
棟	unit, ward
病室	patient's room
看護師詰所	nurses' station
外来診療部門	outpatient department
日帰り手術部門	ambulatory surgery day surgery
外来（診察室）	outpatient clinic
救命救急部	emergency department
救命救急室	emergency room
受付	reception desk
待合室	waiting room
薬局	pharmacy
内科病棟	internal medicine unit (ward)
外科病棟	surgery unit (ward)
整形外科病棟	orthopedics unit (ward)
小児科病棟	pediatrics unit (ward)
産科病棟	obstetrics unit (ward)
婦人科病棟	gynecology unit (ward)
伝染病棟	contagious (communicable) disease unit (ward)
手術室	operating room (OR)
中央材料室	central supply room
回復室	recovery room
分娩室	delivery room
集中治療室	intensive care unit (ICU)
新生児集中診療室	neonatal intensive care unit (NICU)
冠動脈疾患集中治療室	coronary care unit (CCU)
診察室	examination room
処置室	treatment room
検査室	laboratory
リハビリ外来（室）	rehabilitation clinic (room)
レントゲン室	x-ray room
水治療法室	hydrotherapy room
高圧酸素室	hyperbaric chamber
隔離室	isolation room
MRI，PET室など	imaging room

身体の部位の名称（器官図への付録）

脳 (brain)

大脳	brain, cerebrum
大脳基底部	basal forebrain
小脳	cerebellum
小脳基底部	cerebellum basal
前頭葉	frontal lobe
後頭葉	occipital lobe
側頭葉	temporal lobe
頭頂葉	parietal lobe

目 (eye)

結膜	conjunctiva
瞳孔	pupil
角膜	cornea
虹彩	iris
水晶体	lens
毛様体	ciliary body
硝子体	vitreous body
網膜	retina
脈絡膜	choroid
強膜	sclera
視神経	optic nerve

耳 (ear)

鼓膜	tympanic membrane
つち骨	malleus
きぬた骨	incus
あぶみ骨	stapes
半規管	semicircular ducts
蝸牛	cochlea
内耳	internal ear
中耳	middle ear
耳管	auditory tube
外耳道	external acoustic meatus

口腔～喉 (oral, throat)

口	mouth
口唇	lip(s)
舌	tongue
口腔	oral cavity
扁桃	tonsil
咽頭	pharynx
喉	throat
声帯	vocal cord(s)
気管	trachea

心臓循環器系 (cardiovascular)

三尖弁	tricuspid valve
右心房	right atrium
左心房	left atrium
右心室	right ventricle
左心室	left ventricle
上行大動脈	ascending aorta
大動脈弁	aortic valve
僧帽弁	mitral valve
大動脈	aorta
上大静脈	superior vena cava
下大静脈	inferior vena cava
肺静脈	pulmonary vein
肺動脈幹	pulmonary trunk

男性生殖器 (male genital organs)

精嚢	seminal vesicle
前立腺	prostate, prostate gland
陰茎	penis
陰嚢	scrotum
精巣	testis
睾丸	testicle

女性生殖器 (female genital organs)

卵管	Fallopian tube
卵巣	ovary
子宮	uterus
子宮頸	cervix
陰核	clitoris
外陰	external genital
膣	vagina
羊膜	amnion
絨毛膜	chorion
臍帯	umbilical cord
羊水	amniotic fluid
胚外体腔	extraembryonic coelom
卵黄嚢	yolk sac
羊膜腔	amniotic cavity

Measurement　度量衡換算表

● Temperature（温度）

摂氏(℃)×$\frac{9}{5}$+32＝華氏(℉)

華氏(℉)−32×$\frac{5}{9}$＝摂氏(℃)

〔例〕37℃×$\frac{9}{5}$+32＝98.6℉

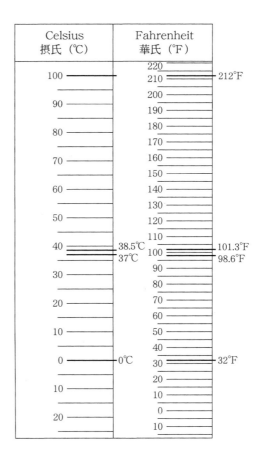

● Length（長さ）　1フィート＝0.3048メートル　1インチ＝2.54センチメートル

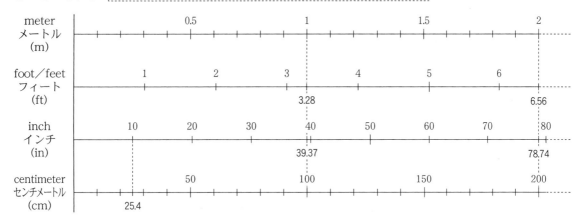

● Weight（重さ）　1ポンド＝0.4536キログラム

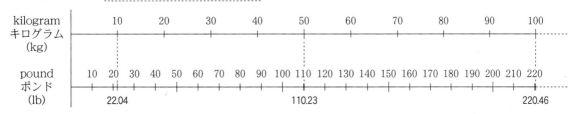

著者紹介

Paul F.Zito

トリニティ大学大学院政治経済分野政治領域修士課程修了。コロラド大学文学部哲学科卒業。スタンフォード大学編集者講座修了。政治学修士。英文PHP誌編集長，九州大谷短期大学教授，イリノイ大学人類学部客員教授，九州女子大学文学部教授を歴任。翻訳者，編集者としても活躍。看護，医学英語に関しては，聖マリア看護短期大学，宗像看護専門学校，久留米大学病院等において教鞭をとる。1993～2006年シアトル居住。2006年より東京在住。

早野ZITO真佐子

国際医療福祉大学大学院医療福祉ジャーナリズム領域修士課程修了。東京大学医療政策人材養成講座修了。青山学院大学文学部英米文学科卒業。コネティカット大学，州立コネティカット大学，イリノイ大学留学。児童文学翻訳家／研究者，短大・看護専門学校・久留米大学病院講師（児童文学，医療英語），翻訳専門学校講師，編集者を経て，1993年シアトルに移住。1994年より医療，看護関連の翻訳，通訳，編集，執筆業。日米の大学，病院と協働で看護／医療研修企画実施多数。2006年に帰国し，その後，帝京科学大学，東京医療保健大学，東京都立大学大学院等で教鞭をとる。また，東京医療保健大学国際交流アドバイザーとして看護学生等の海外研修プログラムを担当。医療福祉ジャーナリストとして看護・福祉・医療分野の取材執筆活動も続けている。著書・訳書に『ルポ 看護という仕事』（日本看護協会出版会），『ナイチンゲールと「三重の関心」～病をいやす看護，健康をまもる看護』（日本看護協会出版会），『ベナー ナースを育てる』（医学書院），『ベナー 看護実践における専門性』（医学書院），『死ぬ権利はだれのものか』（西村書店），その他多数。

ESSENTIAL ENGLISH FOR NURSES
看護英会話標準テキスト　学生版

1996年3月15日発行	第1版第1刷
2001年3月15日発行	第2版第1刷
2005年4月1日発行	第3版第1刷
2016年4月1日発行	第4版第1刷
2018年3月10日発行	第5版第1刷
2024年3月1日発行	第6刷

著者：Paul F. Zito　早野ZITO真佐子©（はやの まさこ）

企　画：日総研グループ
代　表：岸田良平
発行所：日総研出版

本部　〒451-0051 名古屋市西区則武新町3-7-15（日総研ビル）　☎ (052)569-5628　FAX (052)561-1218

日総研お客様センター　電話 ☎0120-057671　FAX ☎0120-052690　名古屋市中村区則武本通1-38　日総研グループ縁ビル 〒453-0017

札幌 ☎ (011)272-1821　FAX (011)272-1822 〒060-0001 札幌市中央区北1条西3-2（井門札幌ビル）	**大阪** ☎ (06)6262-3215　FAX (06)6262-3218 〒541-8580 大阪市中央区安土町3-3-9（田村駒ビル）
仙台 ☎ (022)261-7660　FAX (022)261-7661 〒984-0816 仙台市若林区河原町1-5-15-1502	**広島** ☎ (082)227-5668　FAX (082)227-1691 〒730-0013 広島市中区八丁堀1-23-215
東京 ☎ (03)5281-3721　FAX (03)5281-3675 〒101-0062 東京都千代田区神田駿河台2-1-47（廣瀬お茶の水ビル）	**福岡** ☎ (092)414-9311　FAX (092)414-9313 〒812-0011 福岡市博多区博多駅前2-20-15（第7岡部ビル）
名古屋 ☎ (052)569-5628　FAX (052)561-1218 〒451-0051 名古屋市西区則武新町3-7-15（日総研ビル）	**編集** ☎ (052)569-5665　FAX (052)569-5686 〒451-0051 名古屋市西区則武新町3-7-15（日総研ビル）

・乱丁・落丁はお取り替えいたします。本書の無断複写複製（コピー）やデータベース化は著作権・出版権の侵害となります。
・ご意見等はホームページまたはEメールでお寄せください。E-mail：cs@nissoken.com
・訂正等はホームページをご覧ください。www.nissoken.com/sgh

研修会・出版の最新情報は
www.nissoken.com

日総研

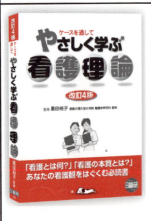

看護理論・看護診断関連書籍

重要なところだけ、短時間でわかりやすく読む 看護理論

成人看護学概論で必要な理論家8人の考え方を

初心者向けにかみくだき、短時間で理論を読める!

［監修・執筆］**黒田裕子**
看護診断研究会 代表

主な内容
- なぜ看護理論を学ぶのか
- 看護理論になじもう
- 重要なところだけ、短時間でわかりやすく読む!
  ナイチンゲール／ペプロウ／ヘンダーソン／ウィーデンバック／トラベルビー／オレム ほか

B5判 180頁
オールカラー
定価 2,420円（税込）
（商品番号 601902）

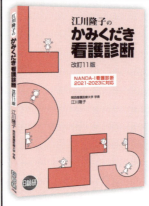

江川隆子の かみくだき看護診断 改訂11版

看護過程の【超基礎】＋【現場で活かす考え方】がわかる

NANDA-I 看護診断 2021-2023に対応

［著者］**江川隆子**
関西看護医療大学 学長
京都大学 名誉教授

主な内容
- 看護診断プロセスの基礎理解
  看護の視点／観察
  情報の整理・解釈・総合
  情報の分析／問題の統合 ほか
- 事例で学ぶ看護診断プロセス
  看護診断過程演習
  全体の事例展開 ほか

改訂11版
B5判 164頁
定価 2,730円（税込）
（商品番号 601928）

ケースを通して やさしく学ぶ看護理論 改訂4版

臨床・看護研究・教育での看護理論の使い方の解説を増強

理論の説明に加え、理論を用いた事例や看護過程の展開を解説

［編著］**黒田裕子**
看護診断研究会 代表

主な内容
- 看護理論を勉強すると何がどうなるの？
- 看護理論をやさしく学ぶために
- 理論家と理論の解説
- 看護理論の教え方 ・年表

増刷出来
B5判 496頁
定価 3,520円（税込）
（商品番号 601817）

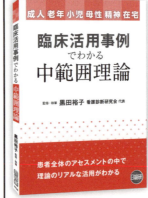

臨床活用事例でわかる 中範囲理論

成人 老年 小児 母性 精神 在宅

がん告知なら危機理論、という固定的・単一的な考え方ではなく、多様な理論の応用がわかる

患者全体のアセスメントの中で理論のリアルな活用がわかる

［監修・執筆］**黒田裕子**
看護診断研究会 代表

主な内容
- なぜ、中範囲理論を学ぶのか
- 成人看護学 ・老年看護学
- 小児看護学 ・母性看護学
- 精神看護学 ・在宅看護学

B5判 192頁
オールカラー
定価 2,530円（税込）
（商品番号 601908）

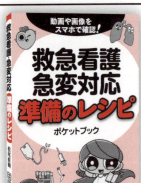

救急看護 急変対応 準備のレシピ ポケットブック

動画や画像をスマホで確認!

チェックリストで症状別に必要な物品などの準備がわかる!

救急・急変場面での急な指示や応援に迷わない!

［編者］**松尾直樹**
独立行政法人国立病院機構
呉医療センター・中国がんセンター
救急看護認定看護師（特定行為研修修了）
他15名の救急看護認定看護師など
救急看護のスペシャリスト

主な内容
- 救急看護・急変対応場面での準備の考え方
- 急性期症状 ・緊急検査
- 家族看護 ほか

A6判 128頁
オールカラー
定価 2,000円（税込）
（商品番号 601927）

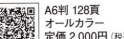

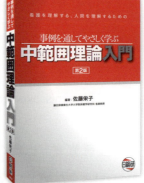

事例を通してやさしく学ぶ 中範囲理論入門 第2版

看護を理解する、人間を理解するための

臨床例での活用方法がわかりやすくなりました

理論を6つ加え、全部で32の中範囲理論を解説!

［編者］**佐藤栄子**
前・藤田保健衛生大学
医療科学部・大学院保健学研究科 教授

主な内容
- 中範囲理論の概説
- 看護の基本姿勢の理解
- 人間の成長発達の理解
- 人間の心理行動の理解
- 病気の過程にある人の理解 ほか

増刷出来
B5判 528頁
定価 3,850円（税込）
（商品番号 600900）

詳細・お申し込みは 日総研 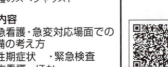 600900 検索

電話 0120-054977
FAX 0120-052690（無料）